Over 1,000,000 Books on Noni Sold

NEIL SOLOMON MD, PhD

NEW YORK TIMES BEST-SELLING AUTHOR, JOHNS HOPKINS CLINICALLY TRAINED PHYSICIAN

THE NONI SOLUTION

THE JUICE MILLIONS OF PEOPLE DRINK
TO ACHIEVE OPTIMAL HEALTH AND WELLNESS

The Noni Solution
Direct Source Publishing
15 East 400 South
Orem, Utah 84058

ISBN 1-887938-44-3

I dedicate this book to the love of my life—my dear wife, Frema, who makes me very happy. To our three special sons and their wives: Ted and Esther, Scott and Florita, and Cliff and Bernadette. And to our precious grandchildren, Scott, Jacob, Bayard, Tessa Grace, and Isabella Rose.

About the Author

Since the 1950s, Neil Solomon, M.D., Ph.D., has devoted his life to the study and practice of medicine. In 1961, he graduated with a medical degree from Case-Western Reserve University in Cleveland, Ohio. He performed his clinical training at the Johns Hopkins Hospital in Baltimore, Maryland. At the Johns Hopkins Medical Institution, he won the coveted Schwentker Award for excellence in research and was a member of the faculty.

While on the Johns Hopkins Medical School faculty, Dr. Solomon spent two years with the National Institutes of Health conducting research in the fields of nutrition, physiology, medicine, gerontology, endocrinology, and heart disease. It was during this time that Dr. Solomon received his doctorate in physiology, with minors in biochemistry and biophysics, from the University of Maryland School of Medicine. For a decade (1969-1979), Dr. Solomon served as the first Secretary of Health and Mental Hygiene in the state of Maryland.

Dr. Solomon is now retired from private practice. He is a consultant to international corporations and to NGO's of the United Nations. Dr. Solomon is a New York Times best-selling author. His interest in preventative medicine and natural healing has motivated him to write and record over a dozen other works about Morinda citrifolia (noni) besides this one.

Some of Dr. Solomon's other educational information on noni includes:

Doctor to Doctor 2nd Edition
What is Noni?
Noni Juice: How Much, How Often, For What

Cancer–How & Why Noni Helps
Happy & Healthy Pets
The Noni Phenomenon

These titles are available from Direct Source Publishing by calling 1-800-748-2996 or by visiting www.nonitools.com.

CONTENTS

Acknowledgments . . . . / 1

The Author's Story . . . ./ 5

Section I: A Singular Fruit

    Chapter 1: The Craze . . . . / 11

    Chapter 2: A Health Revolution . . . . / 27

    Chapter 3: The Science behind the Juice . . . . / 37

    Chapter 4: Power in Numbers: My Survey of 25,000 . . . . / 69

Section II: Noni and Disease from A to Z

    Chapter 5: Arthritis and Pain . . . . / 89

    Chapter 6: Cancer . . . . / 115

    Chapter 7: Chronic Illness . . . . / 145

    Chapter 8: Diabetes . . . . / 165

    Chapter 9: Heart Disease . . . . / 181

    Chapter 10: Infection . . . . / 203

    Chapter 11: Mental Health . . . . / 217

    Chapter 12: Weight Control . . . . / 233

Section III: Noni's Proven Track Record

    Chapter 13: Noni—A Safe Player . . . . / 247

    References . . . . / 256

    Index . . . . / 265

Acknowledgments

To begin, I must deeply thank the 1,227 health professionals who represented 25,314 individuals willing to share their experience with noni juice. You are all what inspired me to write this book.

I also want to especially thank Lois Brown for her expertise in research and editing. In addition, I want to thank the following health professionals for sharing their knowledge of noni with me. They include Dr. Bert Acosta; Alan Bailey; Bryant Bloss, M.D; Dr. Cliff Blumberg; Dr. Carlton Braitwaite; Robert Detrano, M.D; Richard T. Dicks; William Doell, D.O; Dr. Eiichi Furusawa, Dr. Brent Frame; Dr. Charles Garneir, Scott Gerson, M.D; Dr. Ernesto Gomez; Steven Hall, M.D; Dr. Jesse Hanley, the late Mona Harrison, M.D.; Dr. Ralph Heinicke; Dr. Tomo Hiramatsu; Dr. Anne Hirazumi Kim; Dr. Patrick Joseph; Dr. Kay, Dr. Samuel Kolodney; Haruhiko Kugo, M.D; Peter Lodewich, M.D; Dr. Jim Marcoux; Dr. W.T. Meier; John Mike, M.D.; Susan Mike, M.D; Dr. Joel Murphy, Richard Passwater, Ph.D; Orlando Pile, M.D.; Dr. Nathan Rabb, Dr. Nelson T. Rivers; Larry Scott; Keith Sehnert, M.D.; Allen Scheuneman, M.D.; Dr. Rick T. Smith; Gary Tran, D.V.M; Dr. Thomas Velleff; and Mian-Ying Wang, M.D.

Next, I wish to thank Dru and Maeva White, Ken and Mary Roland, Gary and Ann Wilson, Mark and Jo Rose, Floyd and Ann Holdman, and Del and Sylvia Williams for their perspective and genealogical help.

I also want to thank the following for their council and guidance: Kevin and Jenny Baadsgaard, John and Laurie Bentley, Andre and Françoise Blanchard, Dale Brunner, Lil Johnson, Usa Johnson, Susie and Caleb Kwok, Harold and Jesan Ledda, Dayle Maloney, Dave and Dianne Maxwell, Birger Oolvsson, Pat Patterson, Sal and Joan Serio.

Additionally, there are those who provided me with and/or helped me obtain many of the outstanding testimonials I have used in this book and in other of my writing. These people are: Doug Alcorn, Lynn Kathleen Ashcraft, J. Michelle Boykin, Bob and Della Bourke, Carlton and Joycie Braithwaite, Dave and Paulla Castle, Tsai Angela and Lori Chang, E.J. Maki and Siu-Linn Chong, Yalan Lin Chuang, Richard Cooper, Trudy Crow, Robert Dean, Buddy Delaney, Jim Dickson, John Dover, Robert Fechner, Gale, Deborah Gear, Glad Grand International People, Steve and Debra Gray, Marcus and Faith Howship, David Johnson, Gwen Kaese, Marie Mehner and Jack Kelly, Jeanette Komsi, Pat and Sawan Kongpat, Kathleen Gambino Labb, Ivy Way Lee, Sherri and Zachary Lipps, Frances Lowe, Joan L. Mailing, Tom and Elise Markham, Tom Matthews, Paul Miller, Ann Moran, Fay Nicholls-Holt, Ann Olavsson, David and Rosa Olivares, Chuck and Carol Parker, Paul and Margaret Pierce, Dan Ritchie, Joanne Ritter, Helen Rivers, Shannon and Dawn Roland, Karen Rzewnicki, Sal and Joan Serio, Michael Sossin, Terry Sowards, Tom and Manie Thornton, Michelle Titus, Katrina Tran, Jose Miguel Undurraga, Edgardo and Irma Valdivieso, Rob and Janine Witty, Bert and Helga Wolters, Wen Chi Wu, and Joleen Ziegler.

I could not have obtained international testimonials had it not been for the guidance which I received from Brett Barrett, Hector Contreras, John Calvert, Doug Castro, Sun Fu Chong, Cody Day, Lennart Engstrom, Scott Florence, David Garcia, Darrell Ieremia, Eduardo Krebsky, Carsten Marx, Seth Miller, Thorsten Mueller, Craig Richards, Thierry Sorhaitz, Phil Sykes, Edouad Tuairau, Bryant Wadsworth, David Wadsworth, Kenny Wan, Phil Welch, Shon Whitney, and Peter Willden.

I owe many thanks to Jarakae Jensen for sharing his expert scientific and research knowledge about noni; to Pamela Beckham for her gracious willingness to provide whatever assistance was asked of her; to Tom Black, Ben Tyler, Joel Neilsen, Heather Maddison, Andre Peterson, Suzanne Tyler, Blaine Hawkes, Harry Finkelstein, Brett West, and Kathy

Wilson for their input and assistance in numerous matters; to Noni Blues singers Tommy Lyons, Mel Steeple, and Gary Romer for their inspirational songs about noni; to Parveez Shahviri for electronic advice; to McKinley Oswald and his continued confidence and input into the project; to Frema Solomon, M.M.H., my agent and editor who also helped in so many ways.

The Author's Story

All my life, I have been interested in health. From my days as an under-graduate student at Ohio State University to my clinical medical training at Johns Hopkins, I wanted to learn how to improve the quality of life. I was able to do much to this end during my 30 years of private practice specializing in endocrinology and metabolism. Throughout this time, I learned much about conventional medicine. Near the end of my practice, I began learning more about alternative medicine and its potential value in preventative medicine. I have now dedicated myself to the use of com-plementary medicine to bridge the gap between conventional and alter-native medicine. It is for this reason that I am writing this book.

Since 1996, I have investigated the healing properties of a tropical plant, Morinda citrifolia, whose healing properties I believe are making a con-tribution to our general state of health. This plant goes by the common name of noni. I have written several books about noni, but this book is my attempt to pull all that I have learned over nearly a decade of study into one complete work.

My experience with noni has been an interesting one. As I mentioned, I was formally trained as a medical doctor in the curriculums of "conven-tional" medicine. However, during my time as a physician, I always tried to keep an open mind. I have always believed that good health begins with sound nutritional and exercise habits coupled with a strong spiritu-al base. I strongly believe that trying to maintain a life free of excessive stress and emotional turmoil could certainly contribute to good health. However, I never really appreciated how intertwined the body's systems are until I began truly learning some sound practices of "alternative" or "holistic" medicine. I came to understand how feeling good depends on the food we eat, the exercises we do, the music we choose, the prayers we offer, the environment we live in, and a host of other factors. I also learned that some natural-food supplements may strengthen our bodies in the areas where we are the weakest.

Upon being introduced to noni, my reaction was similar to that of many others. I was skeptical. How could a fruit possess any medicinal properties? And the name—a peculiar-sounding name like noni—certainly did not lend credibility to its being a legitimate therapeutic agent. But something triggered my interest. Maybe it was my friend's sincerity that noni was the "real deal." Maybe it was the mystical quality of its history—its origins in South Pacific island cultures spoke of its being used by powerful healers. Or maybe it was my gradually shifting philosophy from that of traditional medicine to one of holistic medicine that pushed me to investigate a little further. Whatever it was, investigate I did.

In the beginning, I talked with a few individuals who knew something of noni. I began digging into the medical literature to see what science knew about noni—where it came from, where it grew, how it has been used historically. I researched what studies had been completed as to its healing value. I even purchased some noni juice from my friends who were distributors for a company that recently began importing it from Tahiti. Most important of all, however, I began to question those who used it to learn what they thought of noni. My preliminary research was intriguing, so I continued.

Next, I took my investigation to anyone who had used noni—homemakers, business people, factory workers, acquaintances, family members, athletes, teachers, secretaries, artists, friends, and anyone to whom they had recommended it. Soon, I had contacted several doctors and other health professionals who were either using it themselves or who were recommending it to their patients. Their feedback once again fascinated me. The data I collected from these first few doctors, which was comprised of feedback from a few hundred patients, revealed some promising initial results. But my skepticism remained.

However, soon more questionnaires, testimonials, and case studies began pouring in by the hundreds. There were stories of dramatic recoveries from cancer, total reversal of chronic pain and fatigue, significant lessening of diabetic conditions, and many other incredible occurrences. I felt the need to randomly sample the doctors and other health care providers to make sure these weren't made up. I did, and I was assured in every instance that the accounts were real.

I was spurred to collect as much data as I could about how people were using noni. I wanted to know the health-related success experienced with its use as well as its side effects and safety. All said and done, I have data from 25,314 noni juice drinkers collected by 1,227 doctors and health professionals. The surveys have shown noni to have value as a food supplement for a wide variety of health conditions from high blood pressure to cataracts to diabetes.

Once noni was introduced to the market, it literally exploded. Millions and millions of bottles of noni juice are sold each year the world over. For almost ten years now I have received extremely positive feedback from hundred of doctors and thousands of noni juice drinkers. This once unknown, strange-looking fruit has now become a household name, and I am very pleased to have been a part of it.

SECTION I

A Singular Fruit

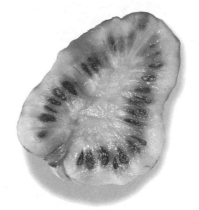

C h a p t e r

1

The Craze

It's ugly, it stinks, and it doesn't taste all that great, yet it's the first thing millions of people reach for in the morning. It's noni, and it has taken the food-supplement world by storm in less than 10 years. Until the mid 1990s, most North Americans had never heard of noni. Now it has become a household word. The first national company to produce and market noni juice recently passed the 1 billion dollar mark in sales.

While noni's physical characteristics are not overly attractive, don't be deceived. For what noni lacks in physical beauty it certainly makes up for in nutritional and medicinal value. Currently, noni is ranked sixth out of the 10 top-selling medicinal herbs in the United States, and the tropical fruit is expected to break the five top herbs soon. But the history behind this strange-looking fruit grown in the tropics is much longer than just 10 years. To really understand noni, we should start at the beginning.

Noni's Story—Past and Present

It all started about 2,000 years ago (as far as historians can tell), when a green, bumpy fruit arrived in Tahiti, Hawaii and other Pacific islands. How the fruit got there is still a bit of a mystery. It is believed it came from the "east" from India and surrounding regions. Perhaps immigrants from the Marquesas Islands purposely introduced noni to Polynesia. Or perhaps it came by accident floating in the ocean with the fruit's brown seeds housed in air sacs that permit the seeds to be buoyant in water. However it got there, noni found Polynesia to be a perfect home. There is ample evidence to show ancient Polynesians (as well as their descendants) used noni extensively for food, cloth dye, and most, importantly for its medicinal properties.

Imagine the village kahuna (or healer) taking a ripe noni fruit in his hands and mashing it to make a poultice for a painful boil or burn. Or envision a wise, Polynesian mother making a cup of noni tea to help soothe her child's upset stomach. Historical documents reveal that scenes such as these were common in older times. Little by little, however, the art of healing became less common. By modern times, some in Polynesia (though not all) had forgotten or never learned of noni's medicinal values.

While the early details of noni's arrival to Polynesia are a little sketchy, how it got to the United States and the rest of the world is not. It all began with dreamers with a lot of ideas but little money. John Wadsworth and Stephen Story had college degrees in food science research, with an emphasis on product development. The problem was… they didn't know what to develop. They had tried a few different products which had failed and consequently they were broke. Then John learned about a fruit called nono, which was used in Tahiti and surrounding areas to treat various conditions, including diabetes. He became interested and was able to get a large gallon glass jar, which was full of a "nono" liquid from some Tahitians who had recently visited Tahiti.

He tested the "nono" liquid on individuals with colds, arthritis, and Type II diabetes. Soon he had enough positive feedback to schedule a trip to Tahiti to find out more. When he talked in detail to natives about the fruit, they always had a story to tell about how it had helped them, a loved one, or a neighbor get better. The illnesses mentioned ranged from cold sores to menstrual cramps, back pain, headaches, cuts and abrasions, diabetes, arthritis, cancer, etc. John also reviewed books that contained recipes of natural remedies written hundreds of years before and handed down from generation to generation. In reviewing the books, he noticed the word "nono" in almost every recipe.

John's first trip yielded so much positive information that he extended his time in Tahiti to further his investigation and see if there was enough fruit to support a large production of "nono" juice. Someone told him that on the Marquesas Islands there was plenty of "nono," and the natives would love for him to gather the "nono" all up. When he checked out the Marquesas Islands, he found that "nono" were mosquitoes and "noni" was the fruit scientifically known as Morinda citrifolia. Eventually, an abundance of noni was found in French Polynesia. In 1995, a company named Morinda, Inc. (now called Tahitian Noni International) was formed, and its goal was to sell noni juice in our modern world as a natural food supplement. This was the first time noni juice had ever been marketed in the United States. Now its use as a food supplement has spread to most of the world.

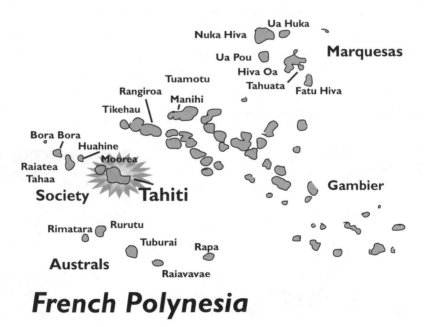

The Noni Basics

Noni, or Morinda citrifolia, comes from the family Rubiaceae. This scientific family has about 80 different species of plants, and only 20 of these species have been identified as having any significant economic worth or being noteworthy in other ways. In fact, the one that stands out as the "queen" of the Morinda genus for its "conspicuous features, its multiple uses, and its supreme ability to distribute itself on seacoasts far and wide without needing human aid" is noni.

The noni plant, which can grow as high as 20 feet, has large evergreen leaves, and its small white flowers sprout at various times during the year. These flowers develop into a bumpy, pitted fruit that is several inches long. Upon ripening, the yellowish-white skin of the fruit thins and turns somewhat translucent. At this point, the usually tasteless flesh becomes unpalatable and takes on an odor (it has been described as having a "rotten cheese smell") that readily seeps through the fruit's skin. Noni has traditionally grown in a wide range of environments, including rocky terrain, fertile lowlands, and sandy areas. The list of areas it inhabits is impressive: it's found in most of the islands of the South Pacific (including Tahiti and Hawaii, the two areas most known for it), Malaysia, Indonesia, Taiwan, the Philippines, Vietnam, India, Africa, Guam and the West Indies (including Puerto Rico and the Virgin Islands). Noni trees produce fruit nearly year-round.

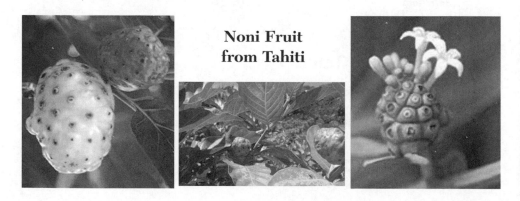

**Noni Fruit
from Tahiti**

From India to Fiji

Noni has been used historically in other cultures besides Polynesia. In India, the fruit of the noni plant was used for cooking and treating diseases. In fact, the noni plant became so popular that it eventually was cultivated as a field crop, with uses for all parts of the plant.

Indian natives also used M. citrifolia for its therapeutic benefits: "Most of the plant is reported to possess medicinal properties. The root is used as a cathartic and febrifuge [fever-reducing agent], and applied externally to relieve pain in gout. Leaves are considered a tonic and febrifuge; they are used as a healing application for wounds and ulcers; the juice of the leaves is externally applied for gout. Fruits are used for spongy gums, throat complaints, dysentery, leucorrhea [abnormal menstrual bleeding] and sapraemia [poisoning of the blood by bacterial putrefaction]."

There are lots of other reports that give us a detailed picture of how noni has been used throughout the years: "In Fiji, the fruit is eaten either raw or cooked. Niue Islanders ate it regularly, and I have been told that the Filipinos made a jam from it, preferring the taste when it was fermented. Other sources report that Australian aborigines were very fond of the fruit. In Burma, the unripe fruits were cooked in curries, and the ripe fruits were consumed raw with salt. Even the seeds were roasted and eaten. Noni fruits are used in Nigeria in the treatment of fever, malaria, yellow fever, jaundice and dysentery. Still other histories report that the over-ripe fruit is stated to be used as an emmenagogue [encourages vomiting], and is recommended... for dysuria [painful urination]. The fruit is sometimes used internally in various preparations for swollen spleen, liver diseases, beriberi, hemorrhage and coughs . . . and as a slightly laxative preparation." These statements are just a smattering of the multitude of historical references to noni and its nutritional and medicinal uses.

"The most significant change was in my mind and my general well being."

David Johnson, a 38-year-old father, was pleasantly surprised with what noni did for him—body and soul.

My name is David Johnson. I am 38-years-old and I have been an insulin dependant diabetic since the age of four. I was diagnosed as an asthmatic 15 years ago. Two years ago I developed angina. Six months later I had an angioplasty to help my heart disease. Three months after that I had a four-bypass open-heart surgery. I have never let my health issues get me down, and I have lived an extremely full life. However, having doctors tell me that there is no hope as a young married man with four young children has led me to times of depression.

About two months ago a friend introduced me to noni juice. I began taking a maintenance dose of one ounce per day. Shortly afterwards, I noticed a number of areas of my health begin to improve. Due to the nature and number of drugs I had to take daily, passing urine was both difficult and painful. The noni juice improved this problem. It also lowered the amount of insulin I required by about 20 percent.

The most significant change was in the area of my mind and my general well-being. It is hard to put into words, but I wasn't depressed, and I felt more uplifted. I increased my noni from one ounce per day to three ounces per day. The benefits likewise increased. My urinary problems became much better, about 60 percent gone. My insulin dosage has now dropped by about 40 percent. My outlook on life is much more positive. And all these improvements came in only two months.

Merging the Conventional and Alternative

The medical world, despite its outward appearance of being on the cutting edge of health advancements, is in general quite sluggish and conservative in its movements. From the time a researcher enthusiastically proclaims "Eureka!" in the laboratory, it may be years before skeptical, cautious and maybe even jealous colleagues are convinced to surrender prior beliefs. Additionally, translating results into practical clinical use where people can actually benefit takes even longer.

Consider a few examples of major changes in the medical world, and the tremendous "lag" time required for the initial discoveries to be translated into practical application. In the early 1980s, an Australian doctor, Barry Marshall, a pathologist at the Royal Perth Hospital in Australia, became convinced that stomach ulcers generally were not caused by stress, as was commonly thought, but rather by a simple bacterial infection. He was so certain he had found the right bacteria that he concocted a potent mix of H. pylori and drank it.

Marshall got exactly what he wanted—a number of nasty peptic ulcers—and more. For almost 20 years, Dr. Marshall and his partner endured incredulity, derision, and outright heckling. Ulcers caused by bacteria? Ridiculous! Everyone knows that ulcers are caused by stress and too much stomach acid.

But in the end, the two researchers won out. Today, there are virtually no remaining skeptics, and overwhelming research shows that ulcers are indeed largely brought about by an overabundance of H. pylori bacteria. Needless to say, there has been a 180 degree turnaround in the manner in which ulcers are now diagnosed and treated.

Another example of the time it takes for medical change is seen in the story of researcher Stanley Pruisiner, a doctor who became extremely interested in the development and treatment of various brain diseases. One of these conditions, called kuru, is a horrific disease commonly found among Fore natives in Papua, New Guinea. These natives practice what Westerners would generally consider disgusting or at least very odd. They eat the brains of their deceased tribe members. Pruisiner's research led him to believe that kuru and other rare human brain diseases were similar to neurological diseases that affect animals, such as mad cow disease.

The standard explanation during this time was that kuru was basically a neurodegenerative condition. In other words, the nerves of the brain simply broke down. Pruisiner had a different idea: he proposed that the nerves ceased to function because of an "infection" by tiny particles of protein called "prions," which lacked genetic material such as DNA. He believed that humans and animals alike could become infected by ingesting prion-contaminated tissues, such as the brains eaten by the New Guinea natives.

Pruisiner's colleagues were extremely skeptical. How could particles that weren't even alive function like live organisms? So stiff was the resistance to his theory that Pruisiner endured almost two decades of being treated as a pariah by the medical establishment. But finally, persistence paid off. Other supporting research began to filter down until finally, Dr. Pruisiner was awarded the Nobel prize for medicine in 1997.

These are just two examples showing how bias, skepticism, and the unwillingness to accept change can significantly slow the process involved in bringing a promising new discovery to the public spotlight. This is particularly true for natural agents (like noni), which typically don't have much of the medical research world's spotlight due to the infatuation with pharmaceutical drugs shared by both the public and the industry alike. Unlike pharmaceutical drugs, most natural products cannot be patented. Because of this, there are extremely few companies that can afford to undergo the rigorous testing required by the FDA (which averages literally hundreds of millions of dollars) before an approval can be granted. This allows a company to make detailed medical claims as to what its product can do. Of course, there is some strict opposition to the rise of herbal and other natural products by some of those in the pharmaceutical drug and related industries. Sad to say, but business is business. Every dollar earned by a natural supplement manufacturer is many times one dollar less for the conventional drug industry. Certainly money and politics play a role in the health laws that are passed, the types of medications that are developed (and authorized by the FDA), and the overall level of care we receive from conventional doctors, hospitals and others. Of course, the industries involved in producing "natural" health supplements are also influenced by money, politics and other hidden agendas.

The point I'm making is that we have the privilege and responsibility to seek out the best of all health-promoting agents and therapies, conventional or alternative. There is good and bad in both the conventional and alternative health worlds. Our job is to investigate what we think are valid, safe and legitimate health promoting products and programs, and utilize them to our benefit.

Noni has literally spread like wildfire in many countries of the world. Its popularity is one of the proofs that this fruit truly does have some unique health-promoting qualities. Things that don't work don't keep selling. They eventually die out. Take for instance the snake oil remedies of the 1800s.

"I noticed significant improvements within a week of taking the noni juice, and after three months all my symptoms were gone!"

Murielle Gauthier from Quebec, Canada, tells about her amazing recovery from an intestinal infection that her medicine was making worse, not better.

In July of 1995, I went to the hospital with an intestinal infection. I was given massive doses of antibiotics. The side effects caused abdominal pain, vomiting, burns on my tongue, and problems with the cerebral nerves.

A long list of consultations with specialists and surgeons only confirmed their inability to find the real problem. They told me I would have to continue taking antibiotics—even if their side effects triggered other symptoms. I was taking 16 different medications without any health improvement.

I went to a naturopath who diagnosed me with candida albicans. After following a treatment of 12 supplements for three months, I noticed a slight improvement. Then I started taking noni juice. After a week, I noticed a significant decrease in my symptoms and an increase in my energy. After three months on noni all symptoms were gone. I feel better now than I did before I was sick. I stopped taking the supplements and medications and now use only noni juice.

I am so pleased with my results with noni juice that I recommend it to anyone with health problems. They will find out what I did—noni juice will improve their quality of life.

Debunking the Snake Oil Myth

Despite recent advances by the natural medicine world, there are some health professionals who still cling to the notion that any agent that is used to remedy not just one, but several health conditions, is simply a fraud, too good to be true. For decades, the "magic bullet" theory that a specific chemical or agent fights mainly one specific disease or symptom, has been drilled into our heads. This theory is the foundation on which the development of modern synthetic pharmaceuticals has been built.

Needless to say, noni advocates find themselves in a quandary. Both the historical and contemporary use of noni suggests that it has been used for a wide array of health problems ranging from chronic arthritis and memory problems to circulatory dysfunction. It could certainly be viewed by some conventional health professionals as a "snake oil" product, touted by overly passionate health nuts bent on convincing the world that the conventional medical world is against them. In fact, I once received an e-mail correspondence from such a doctor. In his comments, he determined that the substantial number of claimed health benefits attributed to noni constituted the "worst case of fraud" involving nutritional supplements that he had ever seen. He said he believed noni was a product whose benefits were unsubstantiated. He thought its use could possibly even be dangerous. In reality, there is not one bit of scientific truth behind his misimpression.

Let's take a quick look at some of the prescription medication currently on the market. There are several anti-inflammatory medications that slow down the body's production of COX 2, a relatively newly discovered enzyme responsible for painful arthritic joints. What many people don't realize is that these same medications are also prescribed for certain types of genetic cancer, and they are also under study for use with Alzheimer's and Parkinson's disease. The obvious link to arthritis, cancer, Alzheimer's and Parkinson's is not obvious to most people at first.

However, each of these seemingly unrelated diseases has inflammation aggravated or possibly caused by the COX 2 enzyme. Should COX 2 inhibitors be labeled as "snake oil" for their wide-reaching effects? No. And neither should natural food supplements such as noni, which has similar COX 2 inhibitory actions.

Researchers usually identify and extract active pharmacological chemicals from plants. And natural supplements conform to standards reflecting specific proportions of those known active agents. This helps ensure that you get an active pill, but it does not totally explain why the herbal remedy, which contains additional chemicals from the plant, works the way it should, or why a crude extract from the whole plant may also work. A good example of this is hypericin, one of the main constituents of St. John's wort, an herb that has displayed powerful antidepressant properties. Initially it was widely believed that hypericin was probably the compound responsible for St. John's wort's antidepressant characteristics. However, it is now believed that an extract of the plant that contains a broader array of constituents than just hypericin has been determined to work even better.

Why? I believe the answer, though difficult to prove, is that most of a botanical's health benefits come from a synergistic effect of several diverse compounds. There are many examples of "natural" products that fit this description. Feverfew, an herb that may effectively prevent migraine headaches, is also used to relieve arthritis pain and respiratory problems because of its anti-inflammatory effects. Even more profound are the almost universal disease-fighting powers of omega-3 fatty acids, commonly found in fish and plant oils, which affect the functioning of nearly every cell of every tissue and organ, and consequently influence a wide array of disorders from brain function to cardiovascular function.

Noni falls into this category. Because of the proposed theory that noni can help the body correct abnormally functioning cells regain normal behavior, its benefits are many and wide ranging. (We'll get to how noni does it in just a moment.) Thus arises the skepticism among those like my e-mail "doctor friend" as to how valuable noni may be.

With the explosion of knowledge regarding natural substances to fight disease, the "magic bullet" theory is slowly fading into the sunset. There are numerous agents that even the most staunch medical conservatives recognize as legitimate in their ability to aid the body in more than one way. Like feverfew and omega-3 fatty acids, these include antioxidants, vitamin C, specific minerals, garlic, ginseng, and others. Historical folk use, as well as modern research and use, have shown noni to be another such agent—a medicinal botanical that can be used for disorders that affect all facets of human health.

"Ten months on 'the juice,' and my victory over osteoarthritis was 100 percent."

Bob Herringer, a 57-year-old, began using noni juice to treat his osteoarthritis, and in so doing enjoyed relief from other health problems as well—including a longtime problem with snoring!

In mid-December of 2000, after a busy holiday weekend, my right knee was swollen and painful—I had obviously overdone it.

I visited my doctor after Christmas. He told me I had osteoarthritis. With my doctor's approval, I decided to treat my condition with noni juice instead of a prescription. I started drinking anywhere from four to six ounces of noni juice each day.

About four months later I was claiming 90 percent victory over the osteoarthritis. The reason it was not 100 percent is, I could still feel a slight surge of pain when going up and down stairs, and I still couldn't kneel on my right knee. However, I was walking as long and as far as I wanted without any discomfort.

I noted other improvements as well. I enjoyed better digestion, more energy, my acid reflux was under control, my athlete's foot problem all but gone, and a winter skin condition did not return. At the top of my wife's list was the fact that after a couple of months on noni my snoring had all but ceased.

After 10 months on "the juice" my victory over osteoarthritis was 100 percent—and continues to this date—some twenty months later.

The Misconception of Approved Equals Safe

There is one last hurdle that many people must clear before they can accept products like noni as a legitimate therapeutic supplement. Because conventional medicines are approved for specific uses by the FDA, many believe they are thus safe and effective to use, while non-approved natural drugs may not only be useless, but also dangerous. It's a common fallacy that natural remedies are used indiscriminately for no valid reasons, whereas conventional drugs are used only for good scientific reasons after being tested and declared safe and effective.

While it's true that the FDA must approve prescription drugs for safety and efficacy before they can be marketed, once they are approved, doctors can sometimes use them for other purposes, tested or not. This is called the "off-label" use of a drug, and the practice is not uncommon. Some reports put the rate of "off-label" use of drugs as high as 50 percent. In other words, five of every 10 prescriptions for a specific drug are used for purposes other than those for which the drug was originally approved. This simply means that potent pharmaceuticals are actually being dispensed with no more proof as to their efficacy than exists for some natural remedies.

> *"The practice of medicine is an art as much as a science. Most of the treatments that doctors prescribe every day are no more 'proven' than the alternative methods they criticize. Accepting unproven and dangerous treatments, while rejecting safer and less expensive natural alternatives, is a bizarre double standard."*
> —*Dr. Alan Gaby, M.D., in* Natural Alternatives.

We must realize that natural remedies aren't necessarily risk-free. Many herbal and natural supplements are potent—if not used with respect they could cause damage to the human body. In addition, there are companies marketing natural supplements who sell their products full of "filler," or who use low quality ingredients. This places both the quality of the product and the integrity of the organization in question.

So, where does this leave noni? In December of 2002, Europe's food commission (equivalent to the FDA in the United States) reported that after intense testing it found "there were no indications of adverse effects from laboratory animal studies on toxicity, genotoxicity, and allergenicity. The Committee considers Tahitian Noni® Juice... as acceptable." While there is a need for more scientific investigation into how noni works, there is no doubt in my mind, due to thousands of years of folk use and the feedback of thousands of modern-day users, that noni is not a snake oil equivalent, a fraud, or a form of quackery. On the contrary—noni is a valuable healing agent that has shown time and time again that its health benefits are many and real.

Chapter Summary Points

- Noni has been used in numerous cultures throughout the world for thousands of years for a wide array of health benefits.

- Noni juice was introduced to North American in the mid 1990s. Since that time it has become extremely popular and is now ranked sixth out of the top 10 top-selling medicinal herbs in the United States.

- Contrary to what some believe, just because people suffering from various health conditions use noni, it is not a snake oil supplement. Much how prescription COX 2 inhibitors are used for more than just arthritis, noni too is used for different problems because of its apparent ability to rejuvenate the body on a cellular level.

Chapter

2

A Health Revolution

We are in the midst of a health revolution. The majority of Americans suffer from health problems resulting from aspects of our modern lifestyles—high-stress occupations, poor nutrition, and far too little exercise. Instead of approaching each day with vitality and an attitude to conquer the world, we typically drag ourselves through the day feeling worn out, tired, and irritable. Sleep does little to remedy the situation, for it is fitful, intermittent, or slow in coming. Many of us cope (though not very well) with aches, pains, sore backs, or stiff necks. We consume inordinate amounts of processed, fatty, and sugar-laden foods; we drink cup after cup of coffee, can after can of soda, and bottle after bottle of alcohol. To cure our ills, we go from doctor to doctor, requesting a three-times-a-day pill that will lift the gloom, lose the pounds, halt the headaches, and hopefully give us a reason to smile.

By now, however, most of us have realized that our current health care system may not provide optimal health care for chronic illnesses or prevention. In fact, more than half of the top 10 diseases that result in death are considered "chronic." And many are preventable. All too often, the premise of the current medical establishment is to use drugs and procedures that often do not cure the problem, but merely mask its symptoms. Though most doctors start their careers with the intent of saving lives, of "making a difference," many become immersed in the paper-work and political games of health-care administrators, the daily routine of prescribing drugs, and the overwhelming task of treating too many patients with too little time.

Top Ten
Killers in the U.S.

Percentages of Deaths per year

1- Heart disease	30
2- Malignant neoplasms (*cancer*)	24
3- Cerebrovascular diseases (*stroke*)	6
4- Accidents (*unintentional injuries*)	5
5- Chronic lower-respiratory diseases	5
6- Diabetes mellitus	3
7- Influenza and pneumonia	2
8- Intentional self-harm (*suicide*)	2
9- Nephritis, nephrotic syndrome and nephrosis	1.5
10- Chronic liver disease and cirrhosis	1.5

Chronic disease has no simple answer. We are learning more everyday, but still much is left unanswered about its causes, and the best treatment. What we do know is that four out of the 10 top killers in the U.S. have a direct link to personal nutrition—heart disease, cancer, stroke, and diabetes. That is incredible in a country where so many health care professionals put such little emphasis on disease prevention through nutrition and exercise. In addition, nearly every single one of the top ten killers has symptoms that go relatively unnoticed for a long period of time. This is another reason why prevention should be considered more important in our medical community than it has been in the past. Think how our lives have changed in the last 100 years.

In 1900, America was at the mercy of germs. Tuberculosis, typhoid, pneumonia, and polio were considered much more terrifying than high blood pressure or elevated cholesterol. A century ago the three leading killers were: 1) tuberculosis, 2) pneumonia, and 3) diarrhea. Those are a far cry from our modern-day top three: 1) heart disease, 2) cancer, and 3) stroke. The most remarkable difference between the old and modern "killers" is that today we are dying of lifestyle choices, not necessarily disease.

Health
Facts

- Every 34 seconds a person in the United States dies from heart disease.
- Smoking accounts for one in 10 cancer cases.
- People who have had strokes are 10 times more likely to have another one.
- Every 20 seconds, a person in the United States has a heart attack.

All of this leads us to ask: "What can I do to achieve optimal health?" The answer, of course, is multifaceted. Now more than ever, many doctors (both traditional and alternative) are encouraging patients to take a holistic approach to health. This is the health revolution I spoke of earlier. Holistic health care includes disease prevention, dietary factors, exercise regimens, nutritional supplements, mental and emotional considerations, and a concerted effort to treat the whole person, not just the sore joints or the hacking cough.

In this holistic approach to health, nutrition plays a vital role. Be it the foods we eat or the supplements we take to complement our diet, our nutritional intake has a profound effect on our overall health. Perhaps that is why when noni emerged on the food supplement scene as a promising medicinal and dietary agent it spread like wildfire. Not that noni is a cure-all or a "magic bullet." It does not "cure" cancer or eradicate other serious diseases; however, if noni supplementation is included in one's holistic health plan, then a happier and healthier life can result.

How, exactly, can noni have such a profound impact on your health? Noni can perhaps help alleviate the pain and stiffness resulting from your arthritis; this, in turn, allows you to go on daily walks and an occasional hike. This increased physical activity leads to enhanced muscle tone and bone strength, which lessens the previously common back aches and decreases your risk of osteoporosis. Meanwhile, you are making more of an effort to eat better, to exercise more, and to watch less TV. After several weeks, you notice that you have more energy throughout the day, you accomplish more at work, and you begin to feel more spiritual, perhaps even attending weekend religious services. Eventually, you wake one day to realize that you feel good: in fact, you feel better than you have in years.

Sound too good to be true? While this example may seem all-too-fantastic to some, it is my belief (and the belief of many other health experts) that it is possible. People using noni to complement a beneficial diet, regular exercise, stress reduction, and an otherwise healthful lifestyle can produce such results. This statement is substantiated by a survey that I conducted over seven years that included the response of more than 25,000 people worldwide who drink noni. This survey showed that 84 percent of those drinking noni for high blood pressure reported a significant drop in blood pressure. Additionally, 69 percent those with cancer reported a significant lessening of their symptoms. Even though I discuss my survey in detail in Chapter Four, I wanted to mention it here to show how people all over the world were enjoying better health, even when they were faced with some of the symptoms of the world's top killing illnesses.

"To me, noni juice is the best natural product in the world. I am living proof that it works!"

Pat Armstrong, a 57-year-old man from Kelowna, British Columbia, was skeptical at first, but the natural components of noni impressed him. After two years on noni, he reports his blood pressure is down, his cancer count has improved, and his arthritis is better.

I am 57-years old and have had some serious medical problems. In 1988 I was diagnosed with cancer. I have had three major surgeries due to my cancer. I also had high blood pressure, my diabetes count was high, and I was stressed to the limit.

Since discovering my cancer it has become important to me to use natural products and to research products before trying them. So, in September of 2000, when my friends introduced me to noni juice, I checked it out. I was impressed to find noni juice is totally natural with over 2,000 years of health benefits. I started taking four ounces of noni per day. Today I am much healthier, physically, and mentally.

After almost two years and a whole lot of noni, I am thrilled to report that my blood pressure is down, my cancer count has improved, my arthritis is much better, and my energy level has increased enormously. Also, I am off two of my daily diabetes pills. I believe noni juice is what has made all of these changes in my life.

To me, noni juice is the best natural product in the world. I have seen so many lives improved with this product. I am living proof that it works. Noni juice has most definitely given me better quality of life, both physically and mentally.

Noni: A Rally Point

The main focus of this book is to help you better understand the nutritional and unique properties of noni in relation to your health. Another theme will be how to effectively incorporate noni into a larger, more encompassing, holistic health plan. That is, a plan that treats the whole body—the mind, the spirit, the emotional and the physical. Since medicine began narrowing its focus on developing drugs as the primary weapon against disease, interest in how the health of the entire body is affected has waned. Early traditional healers (in this case, I mean "traditional" to refer to those native or folk healers who were their societies' principal health care providers before the emergence of allopathic medicine) were very interested in the body as a whole. They viewed the body primarily as an organism whose various systems interacted in a complex and interwoven manner. What happened in the digestive system could very well affect the cardiovascular system; how a person felt emotionally on a particular day could determine whether he or she experienced heartburn that night.

Many Western doctors, on the other hand, have been trained that each of the body's systems is largely self-contained. What happens in the digestive system generally doesn't have much to do with the rest of the organism. Pharmaceutical "medicines" are a focal point in the training and development of the industry. Typically, the primary function of many drugs today is only to mask the symptoms of a particular condition, not to eliminate its cause. As mentioned earlier, because of the innate need for us all to have good health, the research into and development of synthetic drugs and medical procedures has evolved into one of the most lucrative and powerful industries in North America and beyond. It's no secret to anyone that taking one, two, three, or even more pills a day for our various complaints is not only common, but also expensive and acceptable.

Nonetheless, a health revolution is under way. Recent years have seen significant changes in this philosophy. Doctors and health care professionals are beginning once again to return to the basic notion that the body is a complex organism that needs complete, or holistic, care to ultimately achieve greater health. And noni can play an integral part in such a holistic health-care plan.

Where does Noni Fit?

In thousands of individual experiences, I have seen how drinking noni, even in small doses such as one ounce, has helped relieve already existing symptoms as well as helped prevent the onset of others. Since you may be wondering how (exactly) noni could fit into a holistic health plan, let me briefly touch on some of the things noni has been seen to help improve.

Increased energy levels. For centuries, noni was used as a food staple in Polynesian and other cultures, and in times of famine because of its high nutrient content. Current research has verified that noni is, indeed, extremely nutritious. Moreover, modern-day use has shown that a large majority of those taking noni for a specific health condition (other than fatigue or lack of energy) also experience a notable increase in their energy levels. (Later chapters of this book will highlight some of these individuals.)

Relief from chronic and severe pain. Pain, whether a symptom of a known malady or simply chronic in nature, is one of today's most debilitating health conditions. When I was a practicing medical doctor, one of the most common complaints of my patients was that of chronic, bothersome and constant pain. Noni's ability to relieve pain, whether from chronic backaches or from arthritis in the joints, has long been recognized. In fact, Morinda citrifolia carries the self-explanatory title "pain-killer" in various cultures. There is scientific proof that noni can profoundly impact both the severity and chronic nature of various types of pain. (We'll talk more about this in Chapter 5.)

Strengthening of the immune system. This is one of the most intriguing areas concerning noni's amazing health benefits. As previously mentioned, noni was used historically by the various island cultures to treat numerous health conditions. Of course, these people did not understand how noni worked. However, present-day research has discovered that noni possesses the ability to possibly modulate the body's immune functions. For instance, a study conducted by researchers at the University of Hawaii discovered that noni effectively aids the body in fighting cancerous growths by activating the body's production of nitric oxide (NO), cytokines, and other agents that actively seek out and destroy cancerous cells. Other research indicates that noni possesses potent antimicrobial properties (for instance, it has been shown to fight the dreaded E. coli bacteria). This immune-system response is not only evident in humans, but in animals as well.

"Tiger is now playful, healthy, and acting like a kitten!"

Elizabeth Roseborough, from Pittsburg, Pennsylvania, has a 15-year-old cat that became deathly ill. But she says noni juice brought him back to life!

My 15-year-old house cat, Tiger, became deathly ill. His symptoms included frequent vomiting and weight loss. He was down to skin and bones! He had stopped eating solid food and began hiding in dark spots, never playing or socializing. I knew because Tiger was so old the vet would recommend putting him to sleep, so I decided to try noni juice.

Tiger had refused noni juice earlier in the year, so I had to be very clever. I put one teaspoon of noni juice in a teaspoon of half-&-half and mixed it thoroughly. I repeated this twice a day for a week and then added a teaspoon of tuna covered with one teaspoon of noni. This continued for another week, and then I gradually increased everything. I never gave Tiger more than two servings of noni juice a day.

The full recovery took about three months, and now Tiger is back to normal. He is playful, healthy, and acting like kitten!

Chapter Summary Points

- With chronic illness on the rise, we are currently in the midst of a health revolution that is focusing on disease prevention and personal responsibility.

- When incorporated into a well-designed health plan, noni can work wonders in relieving symptoms of numerous disorders, preventing others, and promoting overall improved health.

- A survey of 1,227 doctors and other health professionals receiving data from more than 25,000 noni drinkers found that noni was reported to help decrease the symptoms of a large number of health conditions. This survey has convinced me that noni undoubtedly possesses a variety of medicinal-like properties that modern medicine cannot ignore.

- In general terms, noni can enhance one's life by increasing energy levels, relieving chronic pain, strengthening the immune system, allowing for more physical activity, and helping to prevent the onset of various health diseases and disorders.

3

The Science
behind the Juice

A warm cup of milk. For years it was used as a sleep aid without any idea of why it helped. All your grandmother knew is that it did. In those days if something worked, you used it. With the aid of science we now know that tryptophane, an essential amino acid found in milk, can help induce sleep. It works by increasing the amount of serotonin, a chemical in the brain that acts as a natural sedative. Did grandma know all this? No, she just knew if she couldn't sleep she could warm a cup of milk.

Two thousand years ago did Polynesians know why they ate noni when their stomachs hurt, or why a noni leaf made for a quick-healing band aid? No, they just knew it worked. Today, just as with milk, we have sound theories and concrete knowledge about some of the reasons why noni works. In other words, we have figured out much of the science behind noni juice. It is this "science" I will talk about in this chapter.

Many times people ask me, "How does noni work?" and "How does noni work against so many diseases and health conditions?" These are two great questions, and I hope to answer both.

Noni contains a number of substances—enzymes, vitamins, minerals, proteins, and proxeronine, the precursor to an alkaloid called xeronine—

all which clearly play a pivotal role in maintaining good health. In addition, research suggests that different agents in noni may act in a synergistic manner to produce desirable effects. Of particular interest is how noni exerts its healing action as an adaptogen. Once in the body, the specific components of noni go to the areas in the body where cells are not working properly, and they assist cells in resuming normal function. Much of the research, particularly in the area of cancer, also indicates that ingredients in noni strengthen and modulate the immune system, regulate cell function, and regenerate damaged cells. It is noni's ability to help out on a cellular level that makes it an extremely promising medicinal tool and a candidate to combat a wide variety of health conditions. In the next few pages, we're going to discuss several ways noni provides the body with powerful healing properties. Specifically we are going to discuss nitric oxide, scopoletin, antioxidants, and the xeronine system. In addition to these, there are other disease-specific ways noni helps promote health that we will discuss in the chapters under Section II: Noni and Chronic Illness from A to Z.

Nitric Oxide

Nitric oxide (NO), a substance connected with noni's apparent varied health benefits, may be best known to many as one of the ingredients in smog. In the body, however, nitric oxide is hardly a pollutant. Over the last several years, researchers have uncovered a series of revolutionary discoveries concerning NO and how critical it is to the function and action of a remarkable number of body systems. While noni does not contain nitric oxide, it has been shown in laboratory experiments to stimulate cells from the body to produce it. There have been literally hundreds of research articles appearing in medical journals and text books since the biological role of nitric oxide was discovered in the 1980s—all of these paint a convincing picture that nearly everything the body needs to function correctly depends on the presence of NO. Now that research has shown noni is linked to the body's increased production of NO, we have a good idea how this natural food can help prevent and control various disorders. Dr. Jonathan S. Stamler, a professor of medicine at Duke University, put it quite well when he said, "It [NO] does everything, everywhere. You cannot name a major cellular response or physiological effect in which it is not implicated today. It's involved in complex behavioral changes in the brain, airway relaxation, beating of the heart, dilation of blood vessels, regulation of intestinal movement, function of blood cells, the immune system, even how digits and arms move."

What NO does for You

- It relaxes arteries, and thereby contributes to normal blood pressure levels and heart function.
- It is a potent free-radical scavenger that contributes to lower cholesterol levels and prevents LDL cholesterol (the "bad" cholesterol) from oxidizing.
- It inhibits premature coagulation in the blood, preventing platelets from clumping together into clots associated with strokes.
- It enhances blood flow to the penis, helping boost erections.
- It modulates immune system cells that kill foreign bacteria, viruses, and cancerous cells.
- It has been shown to shrink and destroy some types of tumors.
- It is used by the brain to encode long-term memory and enhance blood flow to the brain.
- It functions as a "messenger molecule" that allows nerve cells in the body and the brain to communicate effectively.
- It aids in the regulation of insulin secretion by the pancreas, helping control diabetes.

Nitric Oxide and Cardiovascular Health

Nitric oxide is heavily involved in many of the body's functions, but most importantly in cardiovascular function as well as in immune system function. However, it has only been recently that the arena of health professionals has come to accept this. The previous incredulity was understandable. Nitric oxide has escaped many physiologists' attention until now because it survives in the body for a mere five seconds or so and because it bears no resemblance to any known biological regulator.

However, just as with noni's popularity, a virtual tidal wave of information regarding NO has come forth, sweeping the worlds of modern medicine in just a few short years and making NO and noni two new potential sources for improving health in broad-spectrum physiological terms. In 1992, nitric oxide was voted "Molecule of the Year" by Science magazine, and consumer health publications began running articles with titles like, "Much Ado about NO" and "Say NO to Impotence!"

How, you may be asking, does nitric oxide help fight hypertension and other cardiovascular conditions? While later chapters of this book will describe this in more detail, let's discuss in simple terms how the heart manages to effectively distribute blood to the entire body. At the center of the cardiovascular system is the heart, which branches off into the aorta, which then distributes the blood to the major arteries, then to smaller arteries, then to arterioles, and finally to the tiny capillaries. The body regulates how these vessels contract and expand to either allow more blood flow or restrict it, depending on the body's needs. For instance, when one is jogging, several areas of the body, particularly the major muscles in the legs, need an increased oxygen flow to produce the needed contractions. On the other hand, if you are outside for extended periods on a cold winter morning, the core organs need increased blood flow to maintain the body's normal temperature.

All of this is achieved via two actions: vasodilation (opening up of the blood vessel—typically the arterioles—so more blood can flow through it) and vasoconstriction (closing of the vessel to decrease blood flow). And it is the smooth muscle rings around the blood vessel that perform these two actions. Imagine the blood vessel as a flexible garden hose that is surrounded by an ace bandage. Tighten the bandage and less water, or blood, is allowed to flow. Loosen the bandage and more can flow freely.

A variety of chemical signals tell your smooth muscle "bandage" to relax or contract. Alcohol, for example, can temporarily relax smooth muscle, allowing blood vessels throughout the body to open up. This is one reason a shot of whiskey on a cold day can make your hands and feet feel warm (though it also increases the risk of hypothermia by not maintaining the temperature of your body's core organs).

On the other hand, when operating properly, the smooth muscle action in your vascular system is anything but arbitrary. It is, instead, a miraculous orchestration with nitric oxide being a principal instrument. This means that nitric oxide created by endothelial cells lining your vessels (which are modulated by noni supplementation) is now known to be a major blood pressure regulator of the body's cardiovascular system.

Nitric Oxide and Cancerous Cells

The body's various defense systems, often lumped together and given the umbrella term of the "immune system," are a multifaceted and complex bunch of processes and agents. Most appreciated in these defense forces are the body's specialized "soldier" cells, such as natural killer cells (NK) that hunt down and destroy enemy invaders such as bacteria, viruses and cancerous cells. We also have a variety of phagocytes, which literally means "cell-eaters," including macrophages that gobble up, dissolve and spit out the few remains of attacking pathogens. There are also what may be referred to as "intelligence" cells that make note of the protein "uniforms" worn by invading cells so that next time they come around, the body's defense systems have designed a neutralizing antibody to render them ineffective.

In the mid 1980s, researchers were able to determine that macrophages—one type of the immune system's "cell-eaters"—had their own form of the enzyme that enables them to manufacture nitric oxide. In the ensuing years, more and more evidence surfaced that nitric oxide may well serve as a sort of "ammunition" that is capable of killing off microbial invaders and cancer cells alike. One good example of this was the published reports of a 1991 study in The Lancet, which showed that 30 grams of oral arginine (which the body uses to produce the NO) given to cancer patients over three days stimulated a 91 percent increase in the ability of their natural killer cells to neutralize cancerous cells.

"Noni juice took care of a potentially serious health problem, naturally!"

Norbert M. DuBois, a 51-year-old man from College Park, Maryland

In 1998 I was getting up to urinate an average of three times a night—a sure sign of a prostate problem in men over 45. When I started drinking noni juice in early 1999, I used it as a general health tonic, not thinking of my irritated prostate. In the early months of 2000, while traveling on an extended job assignment, I noticed I was rarely going to the bathroom more than once a night. Nowadays, I only occasionally go to the bathroom during the night. During my last couple of physical check-ups, the doctors confirmed that I have no prostate problem. It took just over a year, without drugs or any other treatment. Noni juice took care of a potentially serious health problem, naturally!

In October of 1999 I started a new weight lifting program, setting a goal I had never achieved. I wanted to break my 300-pound bench press barrier. Considering I was 'maxing' at 220 pounds, that wasn't an unrealistic goal. My work schedule was the only problem. I was on security detail working 80 plus hours a week, often 28 to 30 days a month. I put myself on a routine of lifting three to four times a week. I usually walked on the days I didn't lift weights. I took three to four ounces of noni juice each morning, one hour before my workouts.

During the Christmas holidays and with the Y2K coming, I worked extra hours without days off. I continued with my workout schedule until finally, in mid-February, I reached my goal! I had two consecutive workouts, bench pressing 302 and 307 pounds. I did this without the aid of any performance enhancing products. The only difference with my diet was my daily consumption of three to four ounces of noni juice. I believe the noni juice fortified my immune system, provided my body with ample proxeronine and infection prevention micronutrients, as well as amino acids and fiber. All of these things combined to help me continue with my crazy work schedule, recover from very strenuous workouts, and reach my weight lifting goal.

I continue drinking three to four ounces of noni juice each morning. Another benefit I've noticed is I rarely catch colds or the flu. All of these benefits from something I thought was just a general health tonic!

Noni stimulates nitric Oxide

What is exciting and promising concerning the use of noni for strengthening the immune system is that recent scientific data has come to light that unmistakably shows that noni stimulates the body's biosynthesis of nitric oxide. A 1997 study from researchers at the University of Hawaii revealed that noni supplementation resulted in a substantial increase in macrophage activity (more than three times the normal). Additionally, when combined with interferon, another of the body's immune function substances, the effect was considerably increased. The researchers go on to recognize that "a series of cytokine assays and NO [nitric oxide] determination demonstrated that noni could stimulate the activation of macrophages. Noni effectively enhanced the production of NO. . ." The notion that nitric oxide, whose biosynthesis is enhanced within the body, can be toxic to cancerous cells is extremely exciting.

Noni's activation of nitric oxide may not be confined to just battling cancer. There are other reports that indicate noni is a potent antimicrobial agent, effectively able to destroy various viruses and bacteria. Most intriguing is the notion that nitric oxide can again act as a deadly form of ammunition against invading pathogens. In some cases, nitric oxide gas interferes with iron-containing molecules crucial to cellular respiration. This kills the invader by poisoning its internal metabolism. Among the common infections that nitric oxide is known to treat by this mechanism are: Salmonella, the bacteria that results in numberless cases of food poisoning each year; E. coli, the infamous bacteria most often seen in food and other contamination cases; H. pylori, the same bacteria discovered by the Australian doctors trying to prove that ulcers were most often the result of bacterial infection; chlamydia, a widespread, sexually transmitted microorganism that results in anything from urethritis to sterility; and last, an overabundance of Candida albicans, which is the most common cause of yeast infection.

The second way nitric oxide neutralizes invading agents is by interfering with the enzymes necessary for DNA replication. By essentially throwing a "monkey wrench" into the actions of these necessary enzymes, nitric oxide can keep infectious agents (as well as many types of cancerous cells) from reproducing, which obviously limits their ability to injure the human body. There are numerous studies indicating that nitric oxide can indeed spur macrophages to disable cancer cells and invading pathogens. One study involving the use of a known carcinogen, showed that only 28 percent of rats given arginine (which the body uses to synthesize nitric oxide) developed cancer, while nearly 90 percent of rats not given arginine developed cancer. In addition, the cancerous growths in the arginine group were most commonly benign growths, while the growths in the control group were of a highly malignant form of cancer. Other studies have repeated nitric oxide's ability to completely destroy various bacteria, viruses and other dangerous microbes.

As early as 1963, noni's ability to fight infectious organisms was shown scientifically. Oscar Levand, a researcher from the University of Hawaii, identified several dangerous pathogens noni was shown to be effective in neutralizing. His carefully constructed thesis states that "the medicinal value of the noni fruit was scientifically confirmed in vitro (in the test tube) by Bushnell and co-workers, who tested 101 Hawaiian plants for antibacterial activity. The juice of the noni fruit was found to be active against three strains of bacteria: Staphylococcus aureus, E. coli and Pseudomonas aeruginosa. Antibacterial activity was also observed against five different strains of enteric pathogens: Salmonella typhosa, Salmonella montevideo, Salmonella schottmuelleri, Shigella paradysenteriae BH and Shigella paradysenteriae III-z. What must also be remembered is that noni can be doubly toxic to invading pathogens. Studies show that it can directly affect various bacteria; additional research suggests that noni stimulates various processes in the body's defense system to further inhibit pathogenic activity.

(ethylthomethyl) benzene
1-butanol
1-hexanol
1-methoxy-2-formyl-3-
   hydroxyanthraquinone
2,5-undecadien-1-ol
2-heptanone
2-methyl-2-butenyl
   decanoate
2-methyl-2-butenyl hexa-
   noate
2-methyl-3,5,6-trihydroxyan-
   thraquinone-6-ß-primevero-
   side
2-methyl-3,5,6-trihydroxyan-
   thraquinones
2-methylbutanoic acid
2-methylpropanoic acid
24-methylcycloartanol
24-methylenecholesterol
24-methylenecycloartanyl
   linoleate
3-hydroxyl-2-butanone
3-hydroxymorindone
3-hydroxymorindone-6-ß-
   primeveroside
3-methyl-2-buten-1-ol
3-methyl-3-buten-1-ol
3-methylthiopropanoic acid
5,6-dihydroxylucidin
5,6-dihydroxylucidin-3- ß-
   primeveroside
5,7-acacetin7-O-ß-D-(+)-glu-
   copyranoside
5,7-dimethylapigenin-4'-O-ß-
   D-D(+)=galactopyranoside
6,8-dimethoxy-3-methyl
   anthraquinone-1,-O-ß-
   rhamnosyl glucopyranoside
6-dodeceno-y-lactone
7-hydroxy-8-methoxy-2-
   methylanthraquinone

8,11,14-eicosatrienoic acid
acetic acid
alizarin
alkaloids
anthragallol 1,2-dimethyl
   ether
anthraquinones
antrhagallol 2,3-dimethyl
   ehter
asperuloside
benzoic acid
benzyl alcohol
butanoic acid
calcium
campesteryl glycoside
campesteryl linoleyl glycoside
campesteryl palmitate
campesteryl palmityl glycoside
campestrol
carbonate
carotene
cycloartenol
cycloartenol linoleate
cycloartenol palmitate
damnacanthal
decanoic acid
elaidic acid
ethyl decanoate
ethyl hexanoate
ethyl octanoate
ethyl palmitate
eugenol
ferric iron
gampesteryl linoleate
glucose
glycosides
heptanoic acid
hexadecane
hexanamide
hexanedioic acid
hexanoic acid

hexose
hexyl hexanoate
iron
isobutyric acid
isocaproic acid
isofucosterol
isofucosteryl linoleate
isolaveric acide
lauric acid
limonene
linoleic acid
lucidin
lucidin-3- ß-primeveroside
magnesium
methyl 3-methylthio-
  propanoate
methyl decanoate
methyl elaidate
methyl hexanoate
methyl octanoate
methyl oleate
methyl palmitate
morenone-1
morenone-2
morindadiol
morindanigrine
morindin
morindone
morindone-6-ß-primeveroside
mucilaginous matter
myristic acid
n-butyric acid
n-valeric acid
nonanoic acid
nordamnacanthal
octadecenoic acid
octanoic acid
oleic acid
palmitic acid
paraffin
pectins
pentose

phenolic body
phosphate
physcion
physcion-8-O[{L-arabinopyra-
  nosyl} (1-3) {ß-D- g-D-
  galactopyranosyl (1-6) {ß-
  D- galactopyranoside}]
potassium
protein
resins
rhamnose
ricinoleic acid
rubiadin
rubiadin-1-methyl ether
scopoletin
sitosterol
sitosteryl glycoside
sitosteryl linoleate
sitosteryl linoleyl glycoside
sitosteryl palmitate
sitosteryl palmityl glycoside
sodium
sorandjidiol
ß-sitosterol
stearic acid
sterols
stigmasterol
stigmasteryl glycoside
stigmasteryl linoleate
stigmasteryl linoleyl glycoside
stigmasteryl palmitate
stigmasteryl palmityl glycoside
terpenoids
trioxymethylanthraquinone
undecanoic acid
ursolic acid
vitamin C
vomifoliol
wax

Scopoletin and Noni

Another of noni's health-promoting agents, scopoletin was first isolated from noni in 1993 by researchers at the University of Hawaii. Following its initial discovery, additional researchers have suggested that scopoletin probably plays a key part in noni's ability to modify blood pressure and help with other medical problems. In 1992, Dr. Isabelle Abbott, a recognized expert in botanical sciences, noted that scopoletin was almost certainly involved in the body's response to noni's effect on hypertension.

As has already been mentioned, scopoletin could act synergistically to contribute to noni's adaptogenic effect. If the blood pressure is too high, it helps lower it; and if it is too low, scopoletin can help raise it. What is interesting is that animal studies have shown that scopoletin, when tested alone, may lower blood pressure to an unhealthy, or hypotensive, level. On the other hand, when tested in a noni extract, scopoletin appears to interact with other agents present in the extract to lower high blood pressure without bringing it too low.

In addition to its cardiovascular effects, scopoletin has been proven to kill a variety of bacterial species, and it is considered fungicidal to Pythium Sp. Anti-inflammatory and histamine-inhibiting effects have also been observed from scopoletin. These two properties help with allergies, skin conditions, and inflammation.

Not only does scopoletin have medicinal properties on its own, but it also binds to serotonin. Serotonin is an essential chemical found in the body's brain and digestive tract. It acts as a neurotransmitter and as a precursor to a hormone necessary for restful sleep called melatonin. Serotonin also plays a role in the body's temperature regulation, hunger, and sexual behavior. Low levels of serotonin contribute to things such as depression, anxiety, and migraine headaches. The lab at the University of Hawaii at Manoa tested the extracts of eight other medicinal plants and none had as dramatic effect in binding to the serotonin receptors as did noni.

"The best thing of all is...I can imagine a future for him!"

Deborah Harr, a mother from Salt Lake City, Utah, tried drugs and therapies with her son for 17 years. Nothing helped his uncontrolable behavior. She considered instutionalizing him before they found noni juice. Now he cleans his room and composes music. What a wonderful change!

For the first two years of his life our son screamed ten hours a day. When he turned two, the temper tantrums started, and by the time he was five we had to put padlocks on all of the cupboards. He kicked holes in walls, and threw toys through walls. If he could find a way to destroy something, he did.

We exhausted all of our savings going from one specialist to another trying to find out what was wrong. One doctor diagnosed him with ADHD. His behavior showed limited improvement with medication, so for the next few years we had to force a pill down his throat. This resulted in two trips to the emergency room for me because he bit me so hard I needed stitches.

Our son is now 17, and ten months ago he was diagnosed on the extreme end of Bi-Polar, manic-depressive illness. We started the recommended drugs in an attempt to control the mood swings and violence, but what we got was little more than a drugged vegetable sitting on the sofa. If he was awake he had a blank stare, but at least he wasn't violent. He didn't like how the drugs made him feel, so he started chewing the pills and spitting them at me. I wondered if the doctors were right about institutionalizing him. But there were good moments with him, too. A few times I had spoken with an intelligent boy inside that hazed and foggy mind. There were moments without violence when I saw an incredible young man living inside the prison of his mind. I knew if we institutionalized him, that incredible young man would be lost forever.

We finally found noni juice and I started giving him one ounce of noni in the morning and one ounce at night. We noticed no change, so we bumped the dose up to two ounces twice a day. There was some improvement, but nothing really exciting until we gave him two to three ounces every six hours of the day. That's when the changes really began! He became a different person—or maybe the person he always was.

Now he is off of all medication. I guess we've been through so much I find it hard to believe it might possibly be over. We have no violent fits, and he even cleans his bedroom. He is getting straight As in summer school, and is composing music and writing a book. The young man, who would only peek out every once in a while, seems to be living here full-time. In the past 30 days he hasn't had one violent rage. The times he feels he might be getting upset he takes some extra noni juice, and that takes care of it.

We may never know the reason for the 17 years of hell we have survived, but whatever the reason, noni juice has been monumental in solving the problem. It doesn't really matter what the condition was, because now we have a solution. The best thing of all is now I enjoy the son we are raising, and I can imagine a future for him.

Noni and Antioxidants

Most medical professionals who are experts in the field of aging agree that damage from free radicals is a significant cause of illness and poor health. Dr. Denham Harman, a professor at Nebraska University, proposed the "Free Radical Theory of Aging" almost 50 years ago. Most of his medical peers ignored his findings for about 20 years. However, in the last few decades, his theories and ideas have been vindicated. Numerous studies since then have proven Dr. Harman correct.

In actuality, there are different ways that free radicals are formed. The first way free radicals may form is when a molecule's weak bonds spontaneously break. The second way is during a body's normal oxidative reaction. The third way of forming a free radical is through radiation, such as ionizing radiation, ultra violet light, etc. Finally, the last cause of free radicals is chemical contamination, especially through human-produced synthetic compounds.

A free radical in the body is an unstable oxygen molecule that must find another electron to make itself complete. So the free radical begins randomly bombarding the animal's bodily cells. When a cell is hit by a free radical, the cell may become more permeable and "leaky," the mitochondria may actually be compromised, or DNA might be damaged.

The damage from free radicals can be countered and prevented by antioxidants. Antioxidants stop free radical damage by donating an electron without becoming free radicals themselves, or they may prevent oxidation from even starting.

There are plant-derived substances on the market that contain high numbers of antioxidants. However, many health supplements are not very potent as antioxidants since they are grown in the same vitamin and nutrient deficient soil as food. Some supplements contain filler or they contain impure plant products. TAHITIAN NONI® Juice is made from fruit that is naturally grown in the unpolluted soils of French Polynesia, Tahiti. It is grown and harvested without the use of harsh chemicals and pollutants.

Tina Ball

Tina Ball, New Zealand Olympic Weightlifting Champion, has achieved 15 percent performance increase since she started drinking noni juice.

Tina competed in the 2002 World Masters Olympic Weightlifting Championship held as part of the Masters World Games, the largest multi-sport event in the world. Tina broke three world records in the 48kg class, Snatch, Clean & Jerk, and Overall Total along with three game records.

Tina has achieved a 15 percent performance increase since she started drinking noni juice. She says, "Although there are many factors that contribute to my sporting success, I feel that drinking noni juice daily cannot be underestimated. It is in my water bottle at every training session."

How Does Noni Compare?

Noni is a powerful antioxidant. In order to combat the potential effects of free radicals and parts of the aging process, the body needs to first prevent oxidization (with an antioxidant), and next, it needs something to rebuild the already damaged cells. Studies show that noni can help do both.

In Table 1, the antioxidant activity of TAHITIAN NONI® Juice is compared to the antioxidant activity of several other well-known compounds often used for their ability to prevent free radical damage. In these results, I use TAHITIAN NONI® Juice as the gold standard, or the substance to which the other substances were compared against.

Antioxidant
Activity (LPO* and TNB**)

Food Supplements Tested	Prevent free radical damage
TAHITIAN NONI® Juice	100% (the gold standard)
Vitamin C	2.8 x Less
Pycnogenol®	1.4 x Less
GSP (Grape Seed Procyanidins)	1.1 x Less

°	LPO = Lipid hydroperoxide quenching activity assay
°°	TNB = Tetrazolium nitroblue, scavenger activity assay
°°°	TAHITIAN NONI® Juice was arbitrarily assigned 100% as the "gold standard," and the potency of other food supplements were tested against it.

The reason for TAHITIAN NONI® Juice's high antioxidant activity may be the result of many different and important compounds found within noni. In particular, I want to talk about these eight:

- Arginine
- Lignans
- Phytosterols
- Glutamine
- Tannins
- Quercetin
- Terpenes
- Nucleotides

The bulk of these are not your garden-variety nutritional supplements that you have heard about all your life like vitamins and minerals. These are very important nutraceuticals.

Arginine, for example, is an amino acid that is credited with relaxing arteries and increasing blood flow. Arginine is also believed to help speed up muscle repair, and with the critical, nitric oxide, it helps in a myriad of functions in the body.

Many researchers recognize tannins, which are polyphenols, as powerful antioxidants. Polyphenols help protect lipids from oxidation, and they have antibacterial and antiviral actions.

Phytoestrogens, such as lignans, have been shown to significantly lower triglycerides (fatty material found in the blood). In addition, this wonderful natural substance promotes hormonal balance, even in women who are going through menopause.

Quercetin, a phytochemical, has antioxidant properties as well as anti-cancer activity. It promotes healthy cells by blocking hydrogen peroxide's (a tumor promoter) effect on intercellular communication.

Plant sterols, or phytosterols like beta-sitosterol, campesterol, and stig-masterol, positively affect the immune system and can reduce inflammation like the synthetic steroids, but without the negative side effects.

Some of the terpenes found in noni are eugenol, beta-carotene and urso-lic acid, all of which are beneficial to the body. For example, beta-carotene is believed to function by helping boost the thymus gland. The thymus gland is known to deteriorate from free radical damage, age, and stress. Beta-carotene provides anti-oxidizing benefits to the gland and in so doing boosts the immune system.

Glutamine is well recognized as a muscle builder. However, its' usefulness goes far beyond that. Glutamine helps to protect muscle protein from degrading in animals, and has been shown to reverse loss of muscle mass from disease, including AIDS.

Nucleotides are cell building blocks and are directly linked to the overall performance of the animal's body and all of its critical organs.

"…there is quite a bit of excitement at the Vosper house!"

Rich Doyle, from Northport, New York, tells the amazing story of a young girl who doctors had diagnosed a quadriplegic and brain dead after a serious automobile accident.

"Mrs. Antoinette Vosper, a nurse, has a 19-year-old daughter who is confined to a wheelchair. Doctors have said the daughter is a quadriplegic, and she is brain dead from severe injuries in an automobile accident. Since the accident Mrs. Vosper and her husband have not been able to sit down to dinner without having to tend to their daughter. She is hooked up to all kinds of monitors, and always needed some attention. After their daughter was on noni juice for five days, they sat down and had an uninterrupted meal for the first time in years. The second night they thought it was simply a coincidence, but after five uninterrupted nights in a row, they felt it was the noni juice. Antoinette reports that the need for suctioning mucous is much less, her daughter's spasms have subsided dramatically, and she is not experiencing her yearly bout with allergies. Since drinking the noni juice, her daughter is trying to speak. At night she goes to bed with a relaxed, pleasant expression on her face—something Antoinette has not seen since before the accident. In addition, the noni juice has helped her daughter immensely with her bowel regimen.

"Recently they took her off the noni, and in two days her former respiratory difficulties resumed, so of course they got her right back on noni juice. Also, Antoinette started taking noni juice for her diabetes. Two weeks ago she was able to stop taking her diabetes medication because she has improved so much.

"I spoke with Antoinette this morning and she reported another extraordinary event. Antoinette said her daughter only makes what she terms "non-purposeful" movements. The other day, while the nurse was blow drying her daughter's hair, her daughter lifted her arm and made a slow, flowing motion—as if she were combing her hair. Needless to say, they have never seen this happen, and there is quite a bit of excitement at the Vosper house."

The Xeronine System—From Pineapple to Noni

The theory behind the xeronine system and noni has a history that really begins in Hawaii in the 1950s with a man named Dr. Ralph Heinicke.

Despite noni's longtime popularity in Pacific cultures as a medicinal agent, until the last half of this century there was little available information, scientific or otherwise, on noni. In the 1950s, Dr. Ralph Heinicke graduated with his Ph.D. and took a job with the Pineapple Research Institute in Hawaii. The company wanted him to commercially isolate the enzyme in pineapple that prevented pineapple gelatin desserts from setting up. Not long after he was given the assignment, Dr. Heinicke figured a way to remove on a large scale the "culprit" enzyme in pineapple. This leftover enzyme extract was called commercial or crude bromelain, and soon the company asked Dr. Heinicke what they could do with this extracted enzyme. In other words, was it worth any money?

This launched Dr. Heinicke into years of research. His initial investigation of crude bromelain revealed little of significant worth; however, he began to receive substantiated reports from other researchers of incredible beneficial medicinal properties associated with the crude bromelain extracts. Physicians were using it to help heal burns, menstrual problems, and other illnesses. Hearing about crude bromelain's astonishing healing properties, the pharmaceutical companies Smith-Kline and Rohr jumped in and wanted to get approval for the marketing of bromelain. To do so, however, they had to purify the crude bromelain to meet FDA standards.

Dr. Heinicke headed the double-blind study required by the FDA for the approval of bromelain. After three months, extensive tests revealed that purified bromelain had lost most of its pharmacological healing properties, even though the crude bromelain worked. A natural course of action for the pharmaceutical companies to take would be to determine why bromelain was ineffective after the purification process. Instead the project was labeled a financial risk, and the companies were dissuaded from further pursuing research that could lead to a complete understanding of how and why crude bromelain worked as a therapeutic agent, when purified it did not.

Thus, for the next 10 years, Dr. Heinicke continued his search for the secret behind crude bromelain and its mysterious constituents. The data was obvious—crude bromelain contained an unknown active ingredient that was destroyed in the purification process. But Dr. Heinicke wanted to know exactly what the active ingredient was. He consulted with Gus Martin, the research director for a company that had meanwhile developed a bromelain tablet product. He and his company provided Dr. Heinicke (and others) with some groundwork data to further pursue the secrets behind bromelain. Dr. Heinicke also worked with Dr. Gerald Klein, who possessed extensive experience with burn patients in World War II, and who had been using crude bromelain to miraculously treat burns.

Finally in 1974, Dr. Heinicke determined that a substance he had unknowingly isolated twenty years earlier from bromelain and which he had regarded as simply an annoying contaminant was perhaps the key to understanding why unpurified bromelain demonstrated pharmacological properties and purified bromelain did not. As it turned out, he discovered this substance was an alkaloid he called xeronine. Alkaloids are an important type of plant chemical that often can have pharmacological properties. He called this alkaloid xeronine because it could be reduced to a dry crystalline structure (therefore the Latin prefix "Xero" meaning dry) and because it had an alkaline nature (therefore the suffix "ine"). Thus the name xeronine (or dry alkaloid) was born.

Through his intensive research, Dr. Heinicke concluded that xeronine regulates the rigidity and shape of specific cell proteins. Xeronine was formed in the body by the combination of a precursor Dr. Heinicke called "proxeronine" and an enzyme named proxeroninase.

Needless to say, Dr. Heinicke was extremely excited at the discovery of this potentially valuable substance. However, what Dr. Heinicke didn't have was the money nor the interest at his current company to further the project. He later took a job with a Japanese company that was interested in his work. While there, he kept in touch with researchers in Hawaii working with pineapple. During three decades, Dr. Heinicke saw the pineapple grown in Hawaii lose many of its nutrients and special enzymes. In fact, he observed that in 1985, 300 milligrams of commercial bromelain from pineapple could not produce the physiological actions that 17 milligrams of commercial bromelain from 1954 could produce. The activity was reduced by about 95 percent. The synthetic fertilization methods with which pineapple growers had grown millions of pounds of fruit over the years had literally changed the chemical make up of the fruit.

He therefore researched other plants that possibly had large quantities of xeronine and proxeronine, the two phytochemicals that had made commercial bromelain from pineapple so valuable. In his search, he learned of noni and found that it contained even more proxeronine and xeronine than pineapple from the 1950s contained. In fact, noni contained up to 40 times more proxeronine than ripe pineapple, its nearest "competitor."

However, most of the noni trees on Hawaii had been cut down because people did not like the smell of the ripe fruit.

He concluded there weren't enough noni trees to make it a viable source of xeronine on a commercial scale. Years later, in the mid 1990s, he was approached by some entrepreneurs who had found an incredibly large source of naturally grown Tahitian noni from which they were to make a bottled juice to sell through a company called Morinda, Inc., the first commercial seller of noni juice (now the company is known as Tahitian Noni International).

"At no time did I doubt the claims made for noni juice. I had seen the data that various drug companies had developed on the pharmaceutical efficacy of bromelain. (These data came from the time when the pharmacological potency of commercial bromelain from pineapple was still high.)

"What few people realize is that no other plant product has ever undergone such an intensive and extensive pharmaceutical investigation as bromelain. Pharmaceutical companies generally only publish work that is pertinent to their pending commercial products. Therefore, much of the work on bromelain was never published.

"One drug company in particular, the one that believed that the discovery of the medical uses of bromelain was one of the major medical discoveries in recent times, tested the use of bromelain alone and in combination with other drugs to treat almost every known ailment. Their data showed success in treating such problems as some types of cancer, some types of arthritis, some types of emphysema, some types of senility, some types of intractable infections, some types of diabetes, some types of blood pressure problems—the list went on and on. Therefore I was not at all surprised to hear that drinking noni juice helped with some of these same problems. I

knew that good quality bromelain and noni juice contained the same active pharmaceutical ingredient. Therefore, the almost miraculous results reported for noni were exactly what I had expected."
—*Dr. Ralph Heinicke, pioneer of the xeronine system*

Understanding Xeronine

Dr. Heinicke has a much better picture now of how proxeronine and xeronine function than he did in the 1950s. He believes it all comes down to proxeronine (the precursor to xeronine) being one of the key substances needed for the body to produce xeronine, one of the agents he theorizes is responsible for noni's impressive array of therapeutic abilities. Xeronine, through a series of biochemical processes, serves as an aid in helping abnormally functioning cells resume normal function and assists normal cells in maintaining their normal behavior. Its activity at the cellular level allows noni to benefit the body in a variety of ways, such as helping fight diseases like chronic pain, cancer, arthritis, and list continues.

According to Dr. Heinicke, both xeronine and proxeronine (xeronine's precursor) are found in noni. However, it is the large amounts of proxeronine within noni that are responsible for its medicinal activity. Let's start at the beginning. The basic components involved in the body's biosynthesis of xeronine are proxeronine and proxeroninase (the enzyme required to catalyze the conversion process). There may be various other compounds as well such as vitamins, minerals, protein, antioxidants, and serotonin. The human body usually produces all of these in adequate amounts except for proxeronine, which is found in limited supply. Ordinarily, the small amount of proxeronine the body harbors is enough to conduct the repairs needed. However, if there is a need for more xeronine in a particular organ—such as when precancerous cells are present, or when there is a viral infection—there may not be enough proxeronine to accommodate this extra need. To get additional proxeronine we must rely on Mother Nature's resources. Sadly, as with the case of Hawaiian pineapple, most of our food supply has been drained of its important nutrients. Noni, however, is the exception.

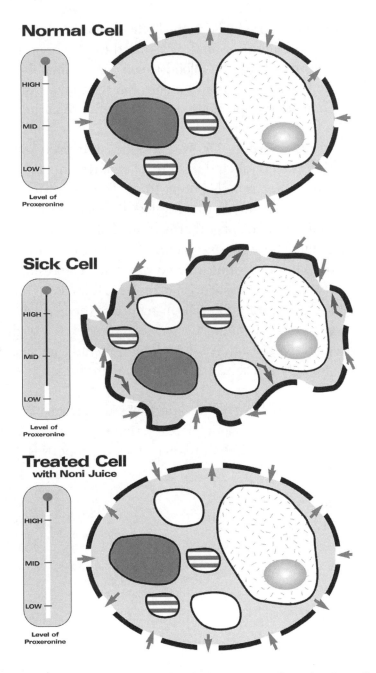

How proxeronine from noni juice helps normalize the function of a "sick" cell.

So, just how is xeronine produced in the body? According to Dr. Heinicke, the liver (which stores proxeronine) is signaled by the brain to release a "shot" of proxeronine into the bloodstream approximately every two hours. The various body organs and tissues can then take from the blood the proxeronine needed to produce xeronine for the repairing process.

At one point in his research, Dr. Heinicke isolated pure xeronine in a crystal form. He then conducted a series of experiments involving mice given tetrodotoxin, an extremely potent toxin. Tetrodotoxin is commonly used in laboratory experiments to kill mice; its injection in mice results in a frenzied, spasmodic display that is immediately followed by death. Dr. Heinicke administered to one group of mice pure tetrodotoxin, and to the other group both tetrodotoxin and xeronine. The results were dramatic, conclusive, and even surprising to Dr. Heinicke. One hundred percent of those given only the poison died as expected—in the usual death throes and almost instantly. Conversely, 100 percent of those given both xeronine and the poison lived! And not only did they live, but they also displayed no outward signs of discomfort or trauma.

Dr. Heinicke repeated the trial several times to test its veracity. Each time, the results were the same. If ever there was a question in Dr. Heinicke's mind as to xeronine's pharmacological properties, there were none after this experiment.

"Within an hour of the first [noni poultice], she had sensation and a pulse in her foot."

Leslee Cook experienced first-hand the effect noni juice has on burns. She says noni saved her foot from being amputated! Elizabeth Jordan, a friend who suggested noni as a poultice, tells the story.

Leslee Cook was involved in a terrible accident. She was treated at the Northridge Hospital in Northridge, California, for several broken bones, and—the biggest problem—large third degree burns on her foot. Four days after the accident, the doctors told her there was no circulation in her foot, and she should prepare for the worst. They would most likely have to remove her foot in order to save her leg.

Since there was nothing to lose, the medical team agreed to allow her to use noni juice as a poultice. I suggested she use noni. The doctors gave us five days to see if the noni poultice would work, but within an hour of the first application she had sensation and a pulse in her foot. Great excitement, to say the least!

After using the noni poultice for a few days the dead skin was peeled away. Her doctor was pleasantly surprised and said it looked like the noni poultice was working. The burns were reduced from third degree to second degree burns. After her accident Leslee began drinking one bottle of noni juice a day. After seeing what noni juice could do, her doctor encouraged her to keep drinking the noni juice. I'm amazed that more doctors don't treat their patients with noni juice.

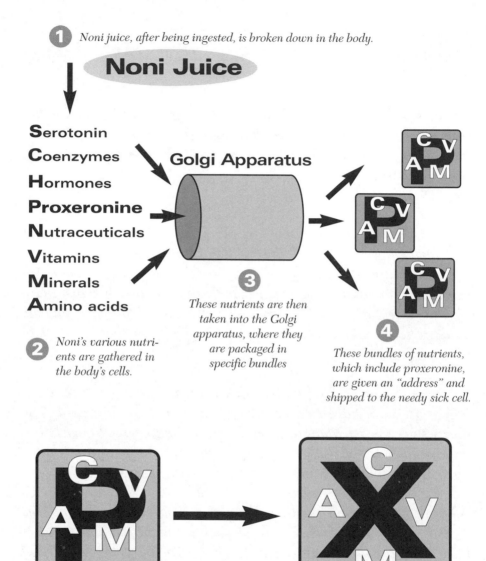

1. *Noni juice, after being ingested, is broken down in the body.*

Noni Juice

Serotonin
Coenzymes
Hormones
Proxeronine
Nutraceuticals
Vitamins
Minerals
Amino acids

Golgi Apparatus

2. *Noni's various nutrients are gathered in the body's cells.*

3. *These nutrients are then taken into the Golgi apparatus, where they are packaged in specific bundles*

4. *These bundles of nutrients, which include proxeronine, are given an "address" and shipped to the needy sick cell.*

5. *When the proxeronine bundles are received by the damaged sick cell, it is then joined with enzymes and other nutrients to form xeronine, which is what the damaged cell ultimately uses to repair itself and regain normal function.*

How proxeronine is converted to xeronine, which is then utilized by the body.

The Golgi Apparatus

The existence of the cell organelle, which is now known as Golgi apparatus or Golgi complex, or simply as "the Golgi," was first reported by Camillo Golgi in 1898. However, the reality of the organelle was questioned for decades, until it was finally seen through electron microscopy. The Golgi apparatus is a complex organelle. It is involved in the processing of proteins and other building blocks that the cell uses to maintain functionality. And while it is not found in every cell in the body, most of the important cells have one.

There is still much to learn about the Golgi apparatus. However, most scientists agree that its principal function is to assemble "packages" of cellular building blocks and ship these various compounds, either to other parts of its cell, or to other cells that need them. It is a fascinating process that may resemble a very effective post office of sorts—each package is "labeled" and "delivered" to the intended cell address, after which the contents of the package are incorporated into the cell and utilized as needed.

Now let's get back to noni. When noni is consumed, its various components are incorporated into the body. One of these components, proxeronine, travels to the cytoplasm of a cell and accumulates in its Golgi apparatus. Within the Golgi, proxeronine combines with the other biochemicals and building blocks the body uses to help maintain efficient and properly functioning cells. These biochemicals would include hormones, proteins, enzymes, serotonin, vitamins, minerals, antioxidants, and various others. The combination of proxeronine with these other compounds is specific and varied, according to the need of the cell to which they are being sent. The Golgi apparatus then assembles the necessary ingredients into a "package," gives it an "address," and delivers it via the bloodstream to the "sick" cell. As the package is opened, the proxeronine combines with the specific enzyme proxeroninase and the two produce xeronine. Xeronine then works with the other biochemicals to create the required adaptogenic compound for that particular cell, allowing the cell to repair and regenerate itself. The limiting factor in this whole process is proxeronine, which Dr. Heinicke believes can be supplemented by drinking noni. The more "sick" or damaged a cell, the greater the amount of noni will be required to repair that cell.

The package of nutrients (including proxeronine) that is bundled by the Golgi apparatus is shipped to "sick" cells possibly in the same way that Rockefeller University biologist Dr. Guenther Blobel has discovered proteins are shipped. In 1999, the Nobel prize in medicine was awarded to. Dr. Blobel, who discovered the "postal system" that allows protein to be sent to cells using a "zip code." This method may be very similar to how proxeronine combines with various nutrients, including protein, to be sent and delivered to a damaged cell. Noni's ability to have a wide ranging relief for symptoms of various ailments, from chronic pain to diabetes to hypertension becomes more understandable once you learn more about Dr. Heinicke's xeronine system, scopoletin, antioxidants and nitric oxide.

"I wasn't feeling good with all the other supplements we were trying, but when I drink just the noni juice I feel great!"

Sharon Boniek eliminated the additional supplements she and her husband were taking when she found them already included in noni juice.

My husband and I drink at least six ounces of noni juice a day. It's the best!

Lately I have been studying many different aspects of nutrition. It seems that many people "in the know" regarding nutrition recommend their favorite supplement. We were taking chromium, digestive enzymes, colon cleansing aids, etc. When I researched what is in noni juice, I found all of the recommended supplements are in there—and in a better form and quality! Why take additional supplements when they're included in noni juice?

Chapter Summary Points

- Noni contains a number of substances—enzymes, vitamins, minerals, proteins, nitric oxide, scopoletin, proxeronine and xeronine—that play a pivotal role in maintaining good health.

- Noni helps stimulate the production of nitric oxide (NO), a valuable substance that provides the body with numerous benefits. Nitric oxide can strengthen the immune system and it has been shown to be instrumental in the lowering of high blood pressure and the improvement of overall cardiovascular health.

- Noni contains scopoletin, which provides other valuable benefits for improved health. Noni has many different ingredients that are high in antioxidant activities. Eight in particular are: arginine, tannins, lignans, quercetin, phytosterols, terpenes, glutamine, and nucleotides.

- Dr. Ralph Heinicke, the pioneering researcher into noni's health-promoting benefits, discovered the "xeronine system," which involves the combination of proxeronine, proxeroninase and other possible biochemicals to form xeronine, which he believes is needed by the body to help maintain normal cell function. Noni contains all of these substances and can help the body increase its supplies of xeronine.

- Noni's success in alleviating various health conditions may be intertwined with the function of the Golgi apparatus. The Golgi apparatus functions as "package" assembler that it then ships to cells that are sick. It is a fascinating process that resembles a very effective post office of sorts—each package is "labeled" and "delivered" to the intended cell address, after which the contents of the package are incorporated into the cell and utilized as needed.

Chapter
4
Power in Numbers:
My Survey of 25,000

Let's pretend you've just come home from the doctor's office where you received a prescription for medication to help with your acid reflux. You get on the internet and read about the studies done on this medication and all of its ingredients. Next, you ask your friend who took the medication what his experience was like and he says, "Awful! The medicine didn't work; it gave me horrible headaches and rashes, so I finally stopped taking it." Are you going to have second thoughts about taking it yourself?

Now let's turn the scenario around a bit. Again you're home from the doctors and doing research on the medication you were prescribed. After you've researched the product, you ask your friend who took the same drug. This time he says, "Awesome. It helped my acid reflux, and I didn't have any negative side effects. I'm going to take this stuff as long as I live." Now how do you feel about taking the product? A lot more secure, I'm sure.

This chapter is your way of asking "a friend" what he or she thought about their experience with noni juice. In the previous chapter you learned about some of the scientific mechanisms in noni that help it promote better health. In this chapter, you will learn what literally thousands and thousands of people who have used noni have to say about it. Then, you will be left to make your own choice about whether this tropical healing juice may be right for you or your loved ones.

"My doctor said, 'Maybe this noni juice is why your MRI looks better.'"

Marie Hakala, who suffers from multiple sclerosis, surprised her doctor with the changes in her health after drinking noni juice.

October of 2002 I had an appointment with a new doctor to try to put some of my physical problems into perspective. I liked this doctor very much. She was very down to earth and not a "drug pusher."

In preparation for this appointment I had three MRIs on my back and one MRI on my brain. In comparing my current brain MRI with the written reports of the previous ones the doctor said there was an improvement. I told her I had been drinking noni juice since September of 1996. She said, "Maybe this noni juice is why your MRI looks better." WOW! I surprised to have a doctor say that. Needless to say, I left her with some information about noni juice.

The earlier MRIs show some lesions, six herniated discs along with some degenerated discs, and some discs that are bulging. The doctor feels these things combined are what account for the problems I have. She reviewed the MRI and suggested I see a neurosurgeon. The bottom line is, in spite of all these things going on in my back I do not regularly take any pain medication. I just keep drinking noni juice, using my chi exercise machine, and going to the chiropractor at least once a month. Some cultures refer to noni juice as "The PainKiller." Noni juice likely works for me because of its anti-inflammatory properties. I resort to prescription drugs very rarely—only if I've tripped, or had a muscle spasm that has pulled something.

Noni juice has also greatly helped in reducing my symptoms of fibromyalgia and arthritis. My husband and I have also noticed that my memory and thought processes have greatly improved since drinking noni juice.

I don't like prescription medications and noni juice has helped me eliminate nine of them. I am very thankful to find something that has gives me much better quality of life without drugs.

Noni's Explosion

As our world becomes "smaller" and more interconnected, information becomes more readily available. Consequently, a legitimate health-promoting agent like noni could not remain a secret forever. And it hasn't.

In 1996, the first commercial noni product, developed and marketed by Morinda, Inc. and called TAHTIAN NONI® Juice, was shipped to the United States. Since then, other noni products have appeared on the market, but Morinda (now called Tahitian Noni International) has approximately 95 percent of all noni sales in the United States and in many other countries around the world. Noni juice has become a food supplement in dozens of countries worldwide.

In fact, TAHITIAN NONI® Juice is the only noni product to pass inspection by Europe's Novel Food Act Committee (much like the FDA in the United States). After rigorous testing, the European committee approved the juice for sale as a novel food in Europe. It concluded, "There were no indications of adverse effects from laboratory animal studies on subacute and subchronic toxicity, genotoxicity, and allergenicity" from the juice.

Countries
Where Noni Juice is Sold

Australia	Indonesia	Philippines
Brazil	Ireland	Puerto Rico
Brunei	Jamaica	Sweden
Canada	Japan	Switzerland
China	Korea	Singapore
Colombia	Macau	Tahiti
Costa Rica	Malaysia	Taiwan
Ecuador	Mexico	Thailand
Finland	Netherlands	United States
Germany	New Zealand	United Kingdom
Hong Kong	Norway	Venezuela

It is no secret that the noni market, both here in the United States and worldwide, has virtually exploded. In fact, recent statistics claim that a bottle of noni is sold every two seconds. This has given me the opportunity to study noni's effectiveness on a large scale. Let me explain how it all began.

25,000 Points of Proof

Shortly after noni products arrived in the United States and Canada, I was asked by a publisher with whom I was working at the time if I had heard anything about a medicinal plant/fruit called noni. I hadn't. Somewhat reluctantly I agreed to research it and see what I could find. A few days after my agreement to investigate noni, I was conversing with some good friends when one of them began describing an amazing medicinal plant she had been using that supposedly possessed a fairly impressive therapeutic arsenal.

"What is it?" I asked.

"Noni," she replied.

I was amazed. Here I had just been given this assignment to find out about some remote tropical fruit, and here was one of my good friends talking about it without any encouragement from me. If I hadn't been initially intrigued by this tropical fruit with the funny-sounding name, my interest now grew by leaps and bounds.

I felt I was on to something. My investigation became more serious, more urgent. Soon enough, I had spoken with enough doctors, health professionals, medical patients, and other individuals who had used noni to treat specific conditions to see that noni was indeed a promising nutritional supplement. As the months passed, I determined to conduct a well-organized and specific survey as to how noni was being used, its success, and its safety and side effects.

My investigations went beyond just the conventional medical realm. I reviewed anything I could get my hands on that might give me better insight into the therapeutic actions of noni. I interviewed doctors, their patients, and others who were currently investigating noni as a medicinal agent. I have spoken with leading herbalists and others in "natural" health fields. I have reviewed popular publications and tracked every legitimate lead regarding the use of noni.

Consequently, since that time I have collected data from 1,227 doctors and health professionals about 25,314 different patients/individuals taking noni. This information has contributed to a formidable database of how noni is currently used.

"I'm not constantly sick like I have been my whole life"

Ellyn Whiteside, a hairdresser, thanks noni for her first healthy winter since she was five-years-old!

As a hairdresser, I am considered high risk for insurance because I touch people. The last time I had insurance was about six years ago. Within the first four months my premiums increased $40 per month. I simply couldn't afford it. I'm so thankful for noni! Thanks to noni, I'm not constantly sick like I have been my whole life. I just experienced my first healthy winter since I was five-years-old. Insurance is still a concern, but since my health has improved so much I no longer worry about not having it.

The Survey Results

To answer the question, "How is noni used today?" I am providing a comprehensive overview of the results of my survey, which demonstrate that noni is used safely and successfully by many people for a wide array of health problems. Let me first give you a few general facts that I found about noni:

- More than two-thirds (69 percent) of 2,188 people with cancer experienced lessening of their symptoms.
- Ninety percent of those who drank noni juice noticed an increase in energy levels.
- Seventy-two percent of overweight noni juice drinkers lost weight.
- Eighty-four percent of those drinking noni for high blood pressure experienced a significant drop in blood pressure.
- Out of 6,828 people with chronic pain who drank noni juice, 86 percent experienced a significant decrease in pain.
- Almost eighty percent of arthritis sufferers reported a lessening of arthritic symptoms (78 percent).
- Side effects among all participants were minimal or nonexistent.

Overall, an astounding 79 percent of the more than 25,000 people who drank/drink noni reported they experienced positive results from the juice. While this survey was not a double-blind study, its results indicate that noni juice does possess some powerful and safe medicinal properties that merit further investigation.

Twenty Nine Conditions

N= 25,314 TAHITIAN NONI® Juice Drinkers
Data collected from 1,227 Health Professionals

Health Condition	# of noni drinkers	% noni helped
1. Allergy	3,198	86 %
2. Arthritis	1,675	78 %
3. Asthma	8,077	71 %
4. Cancer	2,188	69 %
5. CFIDS, Fibromyalgia	3,524	77 %
6. Depression	1,512	80 %
7. Diabetes, Types 1 & 2	5,575	82 %
8. Digestions	3,171	90 %
9. Energy, increased	16,056	90 %
10. Heart Disease	2,158	76 %
11. High Blood Pressure, decreased	1,869	84 %
12. HIV	150	55 %
13. Immune System	3,707	77 %
14. Kidney Disease	3,764	67 %
15. Menstruation	3,798	79 %
16. Mental Acuity, increased alertness	5,543	73 %
17. Multiple Sclerosis	25	52 %
18. Muscle, increased body building	1,216	70 %
19. Obesity, lost some excess weight	5,526	72 %
20. Pain, including headaches	6,828	86 %
21. Parkinson's Disease	25	52%
22. Respiratory Problems, (other than Asthma)	3,857	72%
23. Skin and Hair Problems	877	78 %
24. Sexual Enhancement increased	2,984	84%
25. Sleep, improved	2,025	75 %
26. Smoking, stopped	876	56 %
27. Stress, coped better	6,743	74 %
28. Stroke	1,806	53 %
29. Well-being, felt better	7,879	80 %

During these many years of studying noni, my experience, at times, was a little discouraging and disheartening. Some individuals (excited about promoting noni to their friends, family and others) made outrageous claims regarding noni, making it into a "miracle medicine" that could cure any ailment. In addition, at times I also encountered stiff resistance from acquaintances to the idea that a fruit could provide valuable health benefits. Doctors and other health professionals whom I thought might have an open mind to a new and exciting nutritional supplement have simply dismissed it as an over-hyped fruit juice.

However, on the other hand, my experience for the most part has been inspiring, enlightening, and fulfilling. I have personally seen the dramatic recovery of a woman from the debilitating effects of chronic fatigue syndrome. I have read compelling, honest accounts of recovery. For example, there was the story I received from a Gulf War veteran whose entire family was suffering from various health conditions, yet they all experienced improvement after beginning a regimen of noni use. I was especially pleased to learn of an elderly couple's success in using noni juice to treat cataracts and arthritis. I've had conversations about, received correspondence regarding, and otherwise witnessed the magnificent changes in the lives of individuals who have not only used noni to reverse specific health conditions, but also made the necessary modifications in their general lifestyle to positively affect their health.

I am not the only scientist who has gathered survey data from noni juice drinkers. Another scientist, Dr. Mian-Ying Wang, M.D., several years ago conducted her own clinical survey using noni juice. In Dr. Wang's study, which consisted of 90 patients, 80 percent reported positive results from using noni for a total of 33 health conditions. That means 72 out of 90 people who were sick reported their symptoms lessened after drinking noni. And just like in my survey, the reported side effects were extremely low. In fact, in Dr. Wang's survey, there were no reported side effects.

After reviewing her feedback as well as my own, I have concluded the following:

- Noni helps treat most ailments in a large majority (79 percent) of users.
- Noni usually exerts its effects quickly, with most people experiencing results within days to weeks. (However, most committed to taking noni for six months before deciding how much it helped.)
- Noni is essentially nontoxic, and side effects, if any, are minimal and completely reversible.
- Noni works synergistically with other food supplements and/or medications.
- Noni may help prevent the onset of various disorders.
- Noni is reported to be safe for virtually everyone, including children, pregnant and lactating mothers, and the elderly.

Perhaps one of the most heartening facts that I observed was that so many of the ailments for which noni was effectively used are ailments that are considered chronic and often outside the help of conventional medicine. Patients suffering from lupus and chronic fatigue are often sent home empty handed from their doctors simply because modern medicine knows little about how to help these immune system disabilities. Those with high blood pressure, elevated cholesterol, or painful arthritis often felt that their case was hopeless. My survey showed that thousands of these individuals found hope and health through alternative methods, and particularly through the powerful health-promoting benefits of noni.

"I finally had some control over my health."

Carol, from Palm Bay, Florida, found relief from multiple chemical sensitivity.

I have had MCS (multiple chemical sensitivity) for many years. I react with headaches, pain, confusion, and fuzzy thinking after exposure to chemicals found in products such as perfumes, colognes, cigarette smoke, diesel fumes, glues or aerosol sprays, cleaning products, new carpets, etc.

In August of 1996, a friend who had experienced similar problems introduced me to noni juice. She had been drinking noni juice for a few days and already noticed improvement. I had taken all kinds of vitamins and supplements for years. They seemed to help a little, and I expected the same results from noni juice.

My first day on noni juice I had so much energy I could hardly believe it! I got more accomplished in the next few days than I had in the previous several months. I had started drinking noni juice on a Thursday, and by the time the weekend came I could hardly wait for Monday so I could order two more cases! I never wanted to run out of this stuff.

Over the succeeding months I noticed I didn't get colds or sinus infections anymore. I didn't need antibiotics, decongestants, or anti-inflammatory medications the way I had. My headaches were fewer and much less severe. After eight months on noni my vision had actually improved. I was able to gradually decrease my anti-depressant. I continued to feel better than I had in a long time. If I ever felt a cold or flu coming on I'd take extra noni, along with some other supplements, and by the next day I'd be fine again. I was amazed each time this happened.

I also found I was reacting to chemicals much less severely, and when I did have a chemical reaction I bounced back quickly. After an exposure, instead of getting a severe headache and brain fog for a day and fatigue for several days like before, I'd feel a little spacey for an hour or two and tired for a few hours. Drinking extra noni would speed up the recovery process. I finally had some control over my health.

In October of 1998 my mother had a massive heart attack. I flew to Michigan and cared for her until she died three months later. When I returned to home I had 18 large boxes to unpack, no working vehicle, a neglected business, and of course the grief of my mother's death. I was extremely tired and had little stamina. The tasks before me seemed overwhelming.

I went to my doctor for a complete physical and stress test. My heart was okay but my thyroid levels were low and my thyroid-stimulating hormone was critically low. After an MRI of the pituitary the endocrinologist said my pituitary was not working. He prescribed a new thyroid medication plus oral hydrocortisone. I was reluctant to take hydrocortisone and decided not to fill the prescription. Instead, I increased my noni juice to 16 to 20 ounces a day for about a week. In a few days I started feeling much better. My noni consumption gradually decreased to six to ten ounces a day.

Seven weeks later at my follow up visit my thyroid levels were still a little low but much closer to normal. Test results showed my pituitary was working! I told the doctor I had not taken the hydrocortisone but had increased my noni juice. My baffled doctor tried to explain what had happened, but eventually accepted several booklets about noni juice.

I continue to drink six to ten ounces of noni juice a day. When I'm under stress or exposed to chemicals I increase my intake. I feel I've regained some control over my health and I definitely plan to continue taking noni juice for the rest of my life.

Below is a table of my blood test results.

Thyroid / Blood
test results for Carol Brown

Date Taken	3/4/99	4/15/99	6/28/99*	Reference Range (Normal)
T3 uptake	not checked	37.3	37.4	(28.0 - 41.0)
T4	3.4 (L)	3.4 (L)	4.0 (L)	(4.5 - 12.0)
FTI	1.2 (L)	1.3 (L)	1.5 (L)	(1.6 - 3.7)
TSH	0.05 (C)	0.03 (C)	13.3 (H)	(0.35 - 5.50)

(L) = Low
(H) = High
(C) = Critical

*After consuming larger amounts of noni juice
(Up to 20 ounces a day for a week, then 6 to 10 ounces a day
after a return of energy and less fatigue was noticed.)

The Placebo Effect

The mind is a powerful thing. Have you ever heard of someone unknowingly getting a "sugar pill" and it actually works to cure his or her ailment? When a medicine is prescribed or administered to a patient, it can have several effects. Some of them depend directly on the medicine's pharmacological action. There exists, however, another psychological effect. This phenomenon is called the "placebo effect," and it occurs when the power of suggestion (from words, medicine, a natural supplement, etc…) is strong enough for our mind to help the body heal. The placebo effect happens with conventional medicine as well natural supplements. For example, if your doctor prescribes you medication for a sore knee and reassures you that it will feel better in 48 hours, when you feel better, was from the medicine or the power of suggestion?

The placebo effect is powerful. In a study carried out at Harvard University, placebo effectiveness was tested for a wide range of disturbances that included hypertension and asthma. Incredibly, 30 to 40 percent of the patients obtained relief from these problems with only the use of placebo. One way to test whether a medication is truly effective is to include in experimentation a placebo control group, or in other words, a group that receives something that looks like the medication but isn't. If the group receiving the "real" medication has a higher recovery rate than the placebo-controlled group, you know the medication is effective.

However, there is another way to test for the effectiveness of a drug without having to do a costly placebo-controlled experiment. Simply use the drug with animals. Since animals do not fall prey to the power of suggestion like humans do, this is a very cost-effective way to know the true value of any health-promoting substance. If a veterinarian gives an animal medication to make it stop itching, there is no way for that vet to tell the pet to stop itching. Either the medication works or it doesn't. The placebo effect cannot occur in animals.

> **"We had read about noni juice neutralizing poison, so we were hopeful."**
>
> **Sharon Boniek and her husband from Michigan, have noticed several health benefits from noni juice, but the most amazing story they have involves their dog Duke.**
>
> *Duke is a sweet little beagle—my companion and best friend. One day he came clomping down the stairs, coughing and weaving. He started acting very strange—frothing at the mouth, and growling at me. I knew he had gotten into some poison. I asked my husband to put him out of his misery because I knew that by the time we could get him to a vet he'd be dead. Instead, my husband said, "Get the noni juice!" We had read about noni juice neutralizing poison, so we were hopeful. We gave Duke about three ounces of the noni juice and*

> *checked on him 15 minutes later. I was astounded—he seemed completely normal! Duke ran to the house looking for his supper. After he ate I thought, "Either he's well, or he'll be dead by morning." In the morning he was his usual happy self.*
>
> *I became a firm believer in noni juice for animals. Duke gets his regularly. I know it takes care of worms and is good for his general health. Even though he is 11 years old, he still runs around like a puppy.*

I would like to let my readers know that I understand my survey of more than 25,000 noni drinkers was not a placebo-controlled experiment of noni. No, it was simply data gathered from a lot of people drinking a lot of noni juice. That is the way much good research begins. I do not claim the survey is anything more than a survey. As a scientist, I know that some of the positive results reported in this survey may very well have been from the placebo effect. However, I also know that a typical placebo effect occurs in about 25 to 35 percent of all patients. Therefore, if my survey is reporting success in the numbers of 80 percent, that is a far cry from the 25 to 35 percent caused from placebo.

In addition, my associate and friend, Dr. Gary Tran, has spent several years treating animals with TAHITIAN NONI® Juice. Remember, animals are immune to the placebo effect. During that time, Dr. Tran has used noni juice with at least 10,000 animals. Using noni juice, Dr. Tran says he has been able to improve his treatment success from 70 to 90 percent, depending upon the ailment. By incorporating noni into his treatment plans, Dr. Tran has reduced his allopathic drug inventory from some 300 various types to a couple dozen.

When I began my research on noni, I was quickly made aware that noni's healing influence wasn't only for humans. One of the very first times I heard about using noni on animals was during one of my first conversations with Anne Hirazumi Kim, Ph.D. I was interviewing Dr. Kim for a book. Dr. Kim is an excellent researcher and has published multiple papers on noni in peer reviewed scientific journals. You'll learn more about her in the chapter on cancer.

In any case, Dr. Kim told me her first experience with noni didn't involve a laboratory at all, but that it all started with a dog's water dish. This is her story:

"Ten years ago I had a dog named Brownie who was very sick. My father suggested I give him some noni juice. I had never heard of such a thing as "noni" before. Intrigued, I gave some noni juice to Brownie, at first putting it in his water bowl. He wouldn't touch it. Then I put my hand in his bowl, and he drank it from my hand. Soon he was drinking more of the water/noni combination than what he previously drank of just water.

Before I know it, Brownie started getting better. I was really shocked. He started running around. He regained his appetite, and he just started looking like his old self again. All I could think was, 'Wow, the noni juice really helped him!' It was this experience that inspired me to become a graduate student in pharmacology at the University of Hawaii so that I could study the biological effects of noni juice."

Since that time, I have written a book about using noni with animals, and I have heard many stories that show how effective noni has been with animals. As a medical professional, I see these "animal success stories" as another proof that while there may be some placebo effect going in with the thousands of individuals that drink noni, there is also something very unique about the fruit itself.

"Noni juice has saved me at least $500 in vet bills!"

Jennifer Rosen uses noni juice to treat her cats' ailments—everything from food allergies and diabetes to abscesses and foot problems.

I have two cats. Tippy is a one-year-old black and white shorthaired female. Pumpkin is a thirteen-year-old longhaired red tabby male. Recently I've had three experiences that have proven to me how effective noni juice can be with animals.

Late last year Pumpkin became very lethargic. He slept in a chair in our sunroom for days on end. When I checked him over I found sores all over his body. The vet said the sores were probably due to food allergies. He prescribed special food and antibiotics for Pumpkin, but I decided to give him a daily dose of noni juice instead. I applied a little noni to his open sores as well. Within a week all the sores cleared up and he was running around like a kitten again.

About six months prior to the food allergy healing the vet did some blood work on Pumpkin. The tests showed Pumpkin's blood sugar level was elevated and he might develop diabetes. The follow up visit was about two weeks after I started giving Pumpkin his daily dose of one ounce of noni juice. After a complete work up on all of Pumpkin's body systems the tests showed Pumpkin's blood sugar level had come down from twelve to eight—a very reasonable level.

A couple weeks ago Tippy developed a big lump on her spine. It felt like it had fluid inside and was very tender to the touch. I applied noni to it and gave her about two ounces of noni to drink for three days in a row. On the fourth day the lump had gone down considerably and was starting to heal.

A couple of months ago Pumpkin came home with the end of his tail bloodied. I applied noni to it for two days and it never bled again. His tail healed perfectly. A few weeks later he came home limping. He hissed and growled at me every time I tried to touch his foot. I put some noni on his foot and gave him at least two ounces of noni to drink. He slept for two hours and was in a great mood when he woke up. I gave him another four or five ounces of noni to drink over the next two days. By the second day his limp had improved considerably, and by the third day he was running around like nothing had happened.

Noni juice has saved me at least $500 in vet bills in just those three incidents—not to mention the trauma my cats would have gone through being taken to the vet. The cost in noni juice was about $30. What a savings!

Noni from A to Z

In the following chapters, I will cover some of these debilitating diseases I researched in my survey, and I will show what science has to say about noni (also known as *Morinda citrifolia*) for particular illnesses. In these next chapters, I hope to give you the information you need so that you can make your own informed choice about whether the noni solution will work for you.

Chapter Summary Points

- In the 1990s I began investigating noni's therapeutic capabilities to see if the claims surrounding it were legitimate. This led to my collecting data about 25,314 noni juice drinkers from 1,227 different medical and health professionals.

- The results of the survey astounded even me. An incredible 79 percent of the 25,000 surveyed noni juice drinkers reported noni was an effective food supplement that helped them lessen symptoms or improve overall health.

- In another clinical survey performed by Dr. Mian-Ying Wang, 80 percent reported that noni helped them improve from 33 different illnesses. In this survey, as with mine, negative side effects were minimal or non-existent.

- One of the most heartening facts I observed was that so many of the ailments for which noni was effectively used are ailments that are considered chronic and often outside the help of conventional medicine.

- While all humans are affected to some degree by the placebo effect, animals are not. Therefore, if a medication or natural supplement is effective with animals, that is a good test of its overall effectiveness.

SECTION II

Noni and Disease
from
A to Z

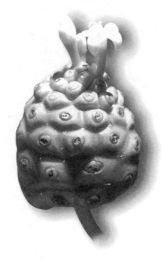

Chapter
5
Arthritis and Pain

Whether it's your back, your knees, your head, or your shoulder, pain is pain. And if you are unfortunate enough to feel pain on a daily basis, you may feel frightened and alone. You may feel helpless. You might even feel as if life is no longer worth living. Being in pain, hour after hour, day after day, rips away your strength, your personality, and even your hope.

This is what happened to Cory—a middle-aged man that looked more like he was in his 60s. His skin was a pale, milky color, though his face was bloated and acne-pocked from the steroids and anti-inflammatory drugs he was taking. Cory was angry—angry at the drugs, angry at his pain, angry at his doctor, but most of all, angry at life itself. But who could blame him? His life was one of constant, severe and widespread pain.

Cory suffered from lupus, an auto-immune disease that manifests itself in many ways. For many sufferers, lupus is more of an inconvenience than a full-blown disease. But for others, including people like Cory, lupus can be excruciatingly painful. After years of various treatments involving all kinds of drugs, numerous hospitalizations, constant fatigue, an almost complete loss of social life, and episodes of deep depression, Cory had been told that his pain was essentially inescapable. This diagnosis, however, was only taking into account conventional treatment. I strongly believe, and have witnessed in others, that significant recovery from chronic pain using a wise combination of alternative and conventional methods is possible. There is hope, and life is worth living.

Chronic pain can result from various sources. And like many health conditions, there are many levels of pain a sufferer may experience. Some of the most common causes of chronic pain are arthritis, auto-immune disorders (such as lupus), and back injury.

But what is chronic pain? Is it a symptom, or is it a disease? Despite being a common complaint, many doctors don't really understand what chronic pain is. Some think that chronic pain is basically the same as short-term "acute" pain. They believe that chronic pain is just acute pain that lasts longer.

That's not true. As we'll examine more closely, chronic pain, though it may originally be a symptom of an underlying condition, usually ends up its own disease. However, chronic pain can be treated, and some doctors have developed rigorous and effective holistic health regimens to relieve pain. When incorporated into a holistic health plan, the exciting food supplement noni has been shown to help those suffering from chronic pain.

"After seven weeks of drinking noni juice I threw away all of my prescription drugs!"

John Russell, from Tuncurry, N.S.W., Australia, tried several different therapies for Paget's disease, but found no relief until noni juice.

For several years I suffered from Paget's disease, the second most common bone affliction after osteoporosis. This disease can cause nerve compression and was the cause of sciatica down my left leg. It became so bad I could not play golf, tennis, dance, or even walk to the next block without feeling a lot of pain. I tried acupuncture, electropuncture, physiotherapy, and deep therapy, but nothing worked.

Then a friend suggested I try noni juice. What did I have to lose? I started to drink it in January 2002, and after about seven weeks of using the noni juice I threw away all my prescription drugs. In May 2002, my Serum Alkaline Phosphate (SAP) reading was down from 350 to 259. I was back enjoying all the activities I loved doing, and I had no pain. Wow!

In addition to helping with the Paget's disease, I have no arthritis pain, and my late-onset diabetes is well under control. Many thanks to noni juice!

How Pain Works

For years, scientists and doctors have not had a complete enough understanding of pain; therefore, pain treatments have usually centered on drugs that partially or temporarily cut off pain without healing its underlying cause. You only need to look at the plethora of over-the-counter and prescription drugs designed strictly to mask pain to know that we have real problems in our society with pain management.

Research and investigative data in the area of pain have revealed it can indeed be reversed through holistic and "natural" means. These treatments have come about because of a fundamental understanding of what pain really is and how it really works.

According to Dr. Dharma Singh Khalsa, author of *The Pain Cure*, pain works within its own nervous system pathway that contains biological "gates" that can be closed to shut off pain. When these gates are closed, the pain is reduced or even eliminated. This concept is often referred to as the "gate theory," and it has brought a much more in-depth understanding that has revolutionized the world of pain management.

A painful impulse usually begins its trip along the pain pathway when you suffer an injury or illness—say, a broken bone. These impulses pass through various "gates" along the way, and will end up at one point in the brain, which then processes and sends the impulse back to the injured area, sensitizing the area and causing inflammation or other localized changes. The sensitizing and inflammation help to protect the damaged area by forcing us to favor it and to help rush healing biochemicals to the area. However, chronic inflammation can eventually magnify the pain or even create new pain through what is called the COX 2 enzyme. This new pain travels back to the brain via the various biological gates—and the cycle once again begins.

As the pain signals come and go, it is easy to see how the cycle can become "engraved" upon the nervous system pathways, causing various elements of chronic pain syndrome to "jam" open the gates of the pain pathway and to magnify the sensations of pain. Eventually these sensations, traveling back and forth and causing more pain, can effectively take on a life of their own. At this point, it is not just a symptom or result of the injury. Instead, it has become its own entity—its own disease.

> **"After being back on the juice, she was running around chasing her tail."**
>
> **Garry and Ingrid Cluley were amazed at the changes in their cats' health when they missed their noni juice for a week.**
>
> *Cats, like humans, have health issues, and I feel it is important to give them noni juice every day. We went away for almost a week, and when we came home I was amazed at how my cats fared without their noni juice.*
>
> *Jasmine has arthritis and was barely able to climb the stairs when we came in the door. Three days later, after being back on the juice, she*

was running around chasing her tail like a kitten again! Jazz also begs and sits pretty well, but was not able to do that until she'd been back on noni for a few days.

Laddie is very muscular cat weighing in at 27 pounds. He has a few extra pounds on him, and as a result is not very active. When we came home he slowly came down the stairs plunked down on the floor and sighed as if to say, "That was enough for me for today." Three days after being back on the juice he was moving around the house, going up and down all three flights of stairs without being out of breath.

The Body's Natural Defense against Pain

The simplest defense against pain is our automatic response to rub an injured site. By rubbing or squeezing the injured area, this sensation sends "touch" signals that outrun the slower "pain" signals. By the time the pain signals arrive at their respective receptor sites, the touch impulses have crowded them out. Other ways the body naturally battles pain is when the brain automatically triggers a release of several chemicals that can flood the brain, giving physical and physiological relief. These substances, referred to as "opiates," not only provide relief from pain signals in the brain, but they also travel to one of the pain "gates" in the spine where they battle the pain-carrying substance-P, trying to keep it from entering the nerves that go to the brain. Some of the more important opiates include endorphins, dynorphins, and enkephalins.

Another way the body battles pain is through the adequate production and utilization of serotonin, a valuable biochemical that helps maintain the proper elasticity in blood vessels, which helps prevent pain common to such ailments as migraine headaches. We'll talk a bit more about serotonin—and its relationship with noni—later in this chapter. If any of these natural defenses are compromised, we experience little, if any, natural relief from pain. Also, there are times when the body's natural inflammation response grows out-of-control, such as is the case with arthritis, which also contributes to chronic pain.

"When I include noni juice with my long workouts I have no muscle pain, and the next day I normally set new health records."

Inge Vabekk, a very active 54-year-old male, uses noni to enhance his athletic abilities.

I started drinking noni juice in April of 2000. I've had several positive experiences with noni, but I'll only share the effects I've experienced related to the sports field.

When exercising, I take 30ml (one ounce) of noni before and after my workout. When I have longer exercise sessions—cycling or hiking for three to five hours—I take more noni once or twice during the workout session. The positive effects I notice when I include noni juice with my workout are quite interesting. Even though I'm exhausted afterwards, I have virtually no muscle pain. And the following day I normally set new records in the health studio. This never happens when I don't take noni juice.

On one outing I tripped and fell, making my ankle very weak. It was so painful I had trouble making it back to the car. I drank about 250ml of noni the rest of the day, and the same amount the next day. The pain was gone! Another time I stretched a muscle in my back. Again, I upped my noni intake for a few days and experienced the same positive results. I'm now taking 200-250ml of noni juice every day—and more if I feel I need it. I strongly feel that my health is worth the cost.

Modern Use of Noni for Pain

A review of the historical literature concerning noni's health benefits reveals that one of its most popular uses in folk medicine was to relieve most types of pain, chronic or acute. From the Eastern medicine healers of Southeast Asia to the Hawaiian kahunas to Caribbean folk doctors, the notion that noni could (and can) effectively treat pain is quite apparent.

There are many modern personal stories about alternative treatment of pain with noni. One chiropractor, Dr. Delbert Hatton, recalls his personal experience with noni and chronic pain. For approximately 40 years, Dr. Hatton suffered from a constant, nagging ache in his lower back from unevenly formed vertebrae. The pain prevented him from doing many of the things he enjoys, and it didn't even let him participate in normal household and yard-keeping duties. After only six weeks of taking noni, his back pain disappeared. He says that after starting to recommend noni to his patients about two years ago, he has had remarkable success in most cases.

One example of success with Dr. Hatton's patients involved a man injured in a traumatic auto accident. He broke several ribs, his shoulder, and his knee. Because of these injuries, he developed severe arthritis in several areas of his body, but especially in his knee. Only days after he started taking noni juice, the patient experienced a dramatic lessening of pain in his knee and a more gradual decrease of pain in his ribs and shoulder. Currently, he is virtually pain-free.

Dr. Hatton provides still another success story involving noni and the treatment of pain. This particular patient broke several bones in her ankle, and consequently suffered from lingering pain and swelling in the area for more than a year and a half. A mere 10 days after starting to take noni the woman reported that both the pain and swelling decreased substantially. Dr. Hatton attributes this to noni's ability to enhance the individual cells' ability to assimilate and utilize the needed nutrients to facilitate repair of diseased or damaged cells and tissue. Dr. Hatton is so enthusiastic about noni's varied health benefits that he declared to me that he would feel confident about noni's chances of successfully treating any kind of health problem, including the very elusive pain-related disease called arthritis.

"My pain level has dropped 85 percent."

Joe Hoerst, a 73-year-old man, is "kickin' high" thanks to noni products.

I have suffered with arthritis for several years, but after I started drinking noni juice six years ago I noticed a great improvement. The same company that makes noni juice came out with a noni extract that has additional natural pain-fighting substances in it. Now the difference is even bigger—and better! I would say my pain level has dropped 85 percent. I am 73 years young and kickin' high thanks to noni.

Arthritis

In Granby Zoo, located 85 kilometers east of Montreal, Canada, is a living, breathing, swinging proof to the effectiveness of noni juice with arthritis. His name is Mumba, and he is a 43-year-old sliverback African gorilla. For years Mumba was the main attraction at Granby Zoo. However, poor Mumba began suffering from such severe arthritis that officials at the zoo thought they might need to euthanize him. Veterinarians had tried all the normal prescription medications, but nothing seemed to work. So zoo veterinarian Marie-Josee Limoges got rid of the medications and decided to go natural. She first added glucosamine and chondroitin sulfate to Mumba's food. Mumba was able to move his arm and get up more easily. By this time, hundreds of animal lovers were sending letters giving their best advice.

"One remedy kept coming up again and again...TAHITIAN NONI® Juice. I tried it first, and between you and me it has a really strange taste, but Mumba took it straight from a spoon," said Limoges.

It was after noni was added to Mumba's diet that zoo officials saw real improvement. The ex-star of the zoo is now the star once more, climbing and moving about his home like his old self.

Why did noni help Mumba? Can natural aids really help decrease the debilitating condition of chronic pain, specifically arthritis? Before I answer these questions in full, let's take a brief look at what arthritis really is.

Arthritis Facts

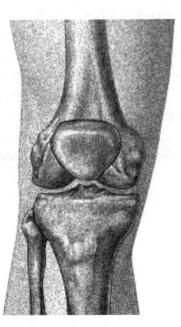

Technically, when you have arthritis it is not your bones that ache, but your joints. However, many times the pain can spread to cause discomfort throughout your entire body. The pain is sporadic at first, and many people may not realize they have arthritis for several months or even years. Only when the pain turns consistent do most people receive a firm diagnosis of arthritis. Other conditions that are related to arthritis are bursitis, tendinitis, systemic lupus, and connective and soft tissue disease. In fact, there are more than 100 different types of rheumatic-like diseases, many causing different forms of "arthritis."

With common arthritis, joints become inflamed and sore from continued wear and tear. The cartilage that cushions the joints degenerates, leaving the raw joints to rub against each other. On the other hand, rheumatoid arthritis, though similar in symptoms, is different in cause. With rheumatoid arthritis the body's immune system begins attacking the body tissues, especially around the joints. Many times there is a red, painful lump located around the rheumatoid joints. Other symptoms are fever, weight loss, stiffness, and loss of energy.

For many years scientists believed that common arthritis has been around for thousands of years, while rheumatoid arthritis was a byproduct of modern civilization. However, recent evidence shows that rheumatoid arthritis is also an ancient disease. After studying the fossil remains of many different cultures, Mexican researchers have concluded that rheumatoid arthritis existed long before European medicine officially recognized it in the 1800s.

These researchers claim that the well-preserved remains of Roman emperor Constantine IX, who lived from 980 to 1055, show he suffered from rheumatoid arthritis. In addition, abnormalities identical to those seen in rheumatoid arthritis have been found in skeletons of Native Americans buried along the Tennessee River whose remains date from 6500 to 450 BC. The point these researchers make is that while it was not uncommon for ancient people to contract the disease, it was uncommon for them to have lived long and fulfilling lives afterward. Sadly, many died young. Gratefully things have changed.

Types of Arthritis-related Diseases

- **Osteoarthritis**—The most common form of arthritis. It affects the cartilage. Over time, the wear and tear of your bones rubbing together dries out the cartilage, making it crack and deteriorate.

- **Ankylosing Spondylitis**—An autoimmune condition in which your body's own antibodies attack healthy cells. It is most commonly seen in young men, and eventually results in the vertebrae fusing together.

- **Bursitis and Tendonitis**—The most common forms of soft tissue rheumatic syndromes, usually caused by the sudden overuse of a joint.

- **Gout**—Occurs when too much uric acid, a waste product in the urea (urine) formation cycle, is either overproduced, underexcreted, or both.

- **Infectious Arthritis**—Many forms of bacteria, viruses, and fungi can cause infectious arthritis, which is frequently characterized by loss of joint function, fever, and inflammation of one or more joints and (occasionally) chills.

- **Rheumatoid Arthritis**—An autoimmune disease brought about when the body has literally started to turn on itself, with the immune system attacking bodily tissues just as if they were foreign invaders. In its mildest form, rheumatoid arthritis is characterized by joint discomfort; in its most serious form it can cause extreme pain, deformed joints and harm organ systems.

Inflammation and the COX 2 Connection

The common link to many of the painful, arthritis-related diseases is inflammation. While the body's inflammation response is meant to help the healing process by signaling to the brain to send special biochemicals (including enzymes) to the injured area, it can turn problematic. The COX 2 enzyme, an enzyme that is closely associated with inflammation, is a relatively new subject in the area of pain management.

Enzymes are proteins that speed up or slow down virtually every biological and chemical reaction there is in the human body. Some of the more common enzymes deal with the human body's digestive system, such as the enzymes found in saliva and stomach juice, which help in the breakdown of food into nutrients. However, there are many more enzymes than just digestive enzymes at work in the body.

For a moment let's focus on just two specific enzymes—COX 1 and COX 2— and what happens when the body's level of these two enzymes is not in balance.

In 1982, the British pharmacologist Sir John R. Vane won the Nobel Prize for his lifelong work with prostaglandins. In his research, which began in the early 1950s, he discovered that the COX enzyme was responsible for the conversion of Arachidonic acid to prostaglandins. These prostaglandins then, in turn, caused painful inflammation. He showed how aspirin stopped the body's production of the COX enzyme and thereby stopped the production of prostaglandins that caused pain and inflammation. However, it was found that people who relied on medications such as aspirin and ibuprofen to control the pain associated with arthritis soon find themselves suffering from a whole new gamut of pain. Non-steroidal anti-inflammatory drugs (NSAIDs) cause gastric ulcers, upper GI bleeding, and colitis. In fact, studies show that half of the people on NSAIDs for pain end up contracting some sort of gastrointestinal problem. For years, however, people put up with the negative side effects of NSAIDs in order to gain some control over the pain. It was the presence of these negative side effects from NSAIDs that spurred researchers into trying to find out more about the COX enzyme.

"I'm convinced noni juice improves my capacity to exercise, and takes away the stiffness."

Margret Haraldsdottir, a 51-year-old pharmacist from Iceland, is delighted with the boost her immune system receives from noni juice.

I've been drinking noni juice for almost four years now and I feel more energetic. My skin is younger looking, my hair is thicker, and I am happier than ever. The best benefit I've noticed is my immune system has improved significantly.

I started to drink noni juice during a period when I wasn't exercising. When I started exercising again I always took a bottle of noni juice with me. I drank one mouthful of noni juice before beginning my routine and smaller sips when I finished. I did not feel the usual stiffness I get when I exercise. One day I forgot the juice. I thought it didn't matter since I'd been exercising for several months without any problems. I was very surprised when my muscles became stiff and sore—the way they did before I started drinking the juice. I'm convinced noni juice improves my capacity to exercise and takes away the stiffness.

My 15-year-old daughter plays soccer. She feels she has much more energy during her practices and games when she drinks noni juice. My 13-year-old son feels the same way. He plays table tennis and played nine difficult games in a tournament last weekend. He sipped the juice during the day and had a great performance.

I believe it is of utmost value to bring knowledge of this wonderful juice to people all over the world.

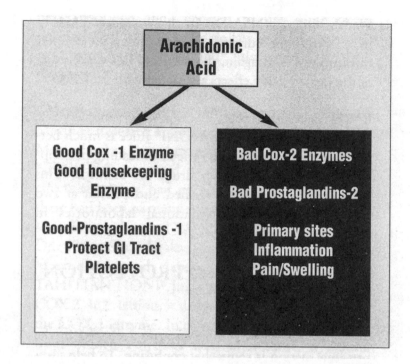

The above graphic visually breaks down the two different enzymes into a simple form. First, the Arcahidonic acid within the body combines with the COX 1 enzyme to create good prostaglandins that protect the stomach and blood platelets. The presence of these "good" prostaglandins gives the body a Protective Factor (PF) that allows continued health in the GI tract. The same Arachidonic acid combines with the COX 2 enzyme to create "bad" prostaglandins that cause inflammation, pain and swelling. The presence of these "bad" prostaglandins gives the body a Misery Factor (MF) that is based upon the presence of pain and inflammation.

The Discovery of COX 2

In 1991, while studying cancer, chemistry professor Dr. Daniel L. Simmons discovered something he was not expecting to find—there was more than just one COX enzyme. It turns out there are two COX enzymes, (and probably more to be discovered later) that differ in terms of genetics, biochemistry, and function. Simply put, COX 1 is "the good COX enzyme" while COX 2 is considered "the bad enzyme." The COX 1 enzyme creates prostaglandins that protect the stomach lining and other parts of the body. The COX 2 enzyme creates prostaglandins that cause inflammation in the joints, muscles and other areas. COX 2 has been compared to a spark plug. The enzyme is the spark, Arachidonic acid is the fuel, and the flame (or burning) of inflammation is the result. In arthritis, this "fire" burns "out of control."

Using Dr. Simmons' research, two large pharmaceutical companies, Merck and Monsanto, created what they called "superaspirins," drugs that selectively inhibit the body's production of COX 2 while leaving the COX 1 enzyme relatively alone. Since that time, these synthetic superaspirins that were supposed to avoid the negative effects of NSAIDs have been reported causing side effects such as rashes, facial swelling, unusual bleeding, and stomach pain. So the search has continued for a natural way to stop the body's production of COX 2, while not significantly affecting the good COX 1 enzyme. This is where noni enters the scene.

Doctor's Recommendation

Dr. Samuel Kolodney is one of the growing number of doctors who not only use noni for themselves but also recommend it to their patients for their ills. "During the past two and a half years many people have reported to me that they recovered from chronic illnesses such as arthritis, high blood pressure, chronic fatigue, joint pain, and diabetes. And the list goes on. However, the first testimonial that truly moved and touched me was from a man with rheumatoid arthritis who proclaimed that noni juice was his 'miracle juice' which had been sent to him by God because it had enabled him to walk when he had previously been confined to sitting because of the constant and severe pain. After two and a half years I still have many miracles reported to me and I witness firsthand many wonderful health changes in people that I have shared noni with.

"My belief in the power of noni to help the body has been fueled both by my personal experiences and those of my clients and the extensive review of scientific literature that I have conducted concerning this amazing fruit. I believe that all edible fruits and vegetables can be healing. I also believe that ounce for ounce noni is the most potent healing food on the planet. Continually encouraged by the results I have seen, I want to make this product available not only to those with specific health conditions, but also to everyone, everywhere."

TAHITIAN NONI® Juice and COX 2

As pharmaceutical companies were in a race trying to patent a drug that would inhibit the bad COX 2 enzyme without destroying the good COX 1 enzyme, Tahitian Noni International was selling millions of bottles of noni juice that has since been proven to be a natural COX 2 inhibitor.

A few years ago, Tahitian Noni International decided to study the effects noni had on COX 1 and COX 2 since there had been so many successful reports from arthritis sufferers who used TAHITIAN NONI® Juice. Dr. Chen Shu, Jarakae Jensen, and others at the Tahitian Noni International research laboratory proved that TAHITIAN NONI® Juice was a selective inhibitor of COX 2. In addition, the juice did very little, if any damage to the COX 1 enzyme. In other words, this natural juice from French Polynesia was, in a sense, a natural "superaspirin" without side effects!

When scientists compared TAHITIAN NONI® Juice's COX inhibition ratio to the COX inhibition ratio of prescription arthritis medications, they found that TAHITIAN NONI® Juice compared "very favorably" to the prescription medications. Yet, TAHITIAN NONI® Juice exhibited none of the negative side effects that the prescription medications are known to cause. Next, researchers compared the COX inhibition ratio of TAHITIAN NONI® Juice to the COX inhibition ratio of over-the-counter NSAIDs. In this category, TAHITIAN NONI far out-performed the over-the-counter medications. And again, the noni did not exhibit any of the negative side effects associated with NSAIDs.

It was concluded that the non-observable adverse effect level of TAHITIAN NONI® Juice is much better than the observable side effects of leading prescription and non-prescription drugs for arthritis. This study was then redone, verified and proven at two more independent, international laboratories in France and Taiwan.

> **"After taking noni juice, the pain is gone."**
>
> **Mona Duncan, a 47-year-old woman, enjoys more energy and freedom from pain.**
>
> *Noni juice has literally changed my life. I couldn't even get in the bathtub because of the pain in my knees. A car accident in 1985 left me with lower back and neck pain. I also have various aches and pains in my fingers and elbow. After taking noni juice the pain is gone. If not for noni juice I would be a miserable aching 47-year-old. Noni has helped me loosen up, feel better, and have more energy.*

Additional Analgesic Qualities of Noni

Richard Dicks, a New Jersey naturopathic educator, had an incredible experience with his son who suffered from a severe bone disease and arthritis. When Richard heard about noni from a friend, he decided to do his own detective work. For eight months, he took noni himself and gave it to his son without telling anyone. The results were astounding. Richard's son's pain dissipated to the point that it was almost entirely gone. How did this happen? Richard attributes the results to noni's effectiveness in cell regeneration and the provision of vital nutrients that help the body battle any chronic condition.

In the last several decades, scientists have studied noni's analgesic qualities with very interesting results. In 1992, Julia Morton, a noted botanist, reported that noni contains terpenes, found in essential oils, which have been shown to aid in cell synthesis and cell rejuvenation. Other recent research reveals that noni contains numerous known essential nutrients, including proteins, amino acids, enzymes, vitamins, and minerals, which may synergistically contribute to noni's ability to fight pain and a host of other ailments.

A laboratory in France conducted a study that showed mice, given a liquid form of *Morinda citrifolia* had increased reaction time to a hot plate. The researchers concluded that the noni helped the mice better deal with the pain from the hot plate.

Other reasons for noni's analgesic qualities may stem from several of its compounds. Noni has been shown to contain scopoletin, which has anti-inflammatory and antihistamine effects, both of which are needed for smooth joint movement. Another component is xeronine, the cell-building substance discovered by Dr. Ralph Heinicke. Xeronine may help prevent and rebuild damaged joint tissue as well as promote a healthier immune system.

"For me, 'noni' meant 'no knee' surgery!"

Michelle Boykin was scheduled for a total knee replacement surgery until she started drinking noni juice. A few weeks later the pain and swelling were gone and the surgery was cancelled. Now, she can run, jump and climb without problem.

In March of 2002 my knee began swelling and causing me some discomfort. The problem continued to get worse, so I made an appointment with my doctor. My doctor sent me to an orthopedic specialist who ordered an MRI of the knee. The visit with the specialist got me a handicap sticker and a surgery date of May 15th.

A friend told me about noni juice. He said he'd heard that people with knee problems were getting good results from noni. I never thought noni juice could help my knee. I knew my friend did not understand. I did not have a knee problem. I had a knee catastrophe!

I started drinking noni juice because I wanted my body to be as strong as possible to insure a speedy recovery from knee surgery. To my surprise, two days after drinking the juice (one ounce three times a day) the swelling in my knee, that the doctors said could only be remedied with total knee replacement surgery, was gone. I was scheduled to visit with one of the leading knee specialists two weeks from the time I began drinking the juice. By the time that appointment came around the swelling and pain in my knee were gone.

I kept the appointment with the specialist just to be safe. After looking at my test results, he recommended a total knee replacement. Then he did the physical exam, and I had no swelling or pain, so he wanted to cancel the surgery. He was curious about what I was doing for my knee. I told him about noni juice. He said that too many doc tors minimize the benefits of these types of remedies. He recommended that I continue drinking the juice, and he felt we might not have to perform the surgery at all. Knowing I was an avid runner, he also warned me that I would not be able to run again. I agreed, if it meant I could keep my knee.

It is one year later, and the only thing I can say is, the doctor was wrong about the running issue. I am pain free, and I run, jump, and climb, with absolutely no problem. They say the natives of French Polynesia named this fruit 'noni', because the word means a gift from God. For me "noni" has also meant "no knee" surgery!

Serotonin and Pain

Recent years have expanded our knowledge of serotonin and the multiple roles it plays in relieving conditions like depression, anxiety, and sleep dysfunction. It achieves these things largely because of the role it plays in the brain and nervous system. Dr. Heinicke's extensive research revealing noni's part in the body's production and proper utilization of serotonin provides us with exciting possibilities as to how noni relieves pain. We know that serotonin, triggered by the brain, tells the nerves that first pick up the pain signal to "calm down," causing the muscles and blood vessels around the injured areas to relax. Your body loosens up, causing the pain to subside and letting you get back to feeling fine.

Dr. Khalsa, author of *The Pain Cure*, also believes that normalizing serotonin levels in the body can help alleviate the effects of pain by more ways than just improving the elasticity of blood vessels. These include raising the brain's pain threshold, promoting healthy sleep patterns, reducing pain-amplifying anxiety, and reducing pain-amplifying depression.

The Link Between Noni and Serotonin

So what's the connection between noni and serotonin? Dr. Heinicke and others suggest that noni works with serotonin in the body to alleviate a number of conditions, including pain resulting from arthritis, autoimmune disorders, and migraines. Remember how the Golgi apparatus "packages" and "ships" important nutrients along with xeronine to damaged cells? There is the strong possibility that in these bundles of nutrients will be found pain-fighting substances like serotonin. As we have already shown, the body uses serotonin to fight pain in a number of ways. But the body can't take advantage of the serotonin if it isn't present within the suffering area. I suspect that one way serotonin becomes available for an affected area is through a smooth-functioning Golgi apparatus that, through the help of the xeronine system, safely and efficiently delivers the serotonin package to the intended target.

> *"My finger was three times its normal size when I applied the noni juice. A few minutes later the pain was gone, and three hours later the swelling was down!"*
>
> *Karen Nguyen, initially used noni juice to help with her son's Hepatitis B, but also found help with some of her own health problems.*
>
> *I purchased noni juice for my son who has Hepatitis B, irritable bowel syndrome, and suffers with depression. After he finished the first bottle of noni juice he no longer pounded on the wall, and he didn't complain about being tired. He expressed himself more calmly.*
>
> *I have used noni juice for many different things. One time I had a toothache, resulting from an old crown. I took one teaspoon of noni juice, held it in my mouth for 15 minutes, and then swallowed it slowly. The pain went away, and my mouth felt fresher and cleaner than ever.*

I used an axe to cut down a tree trunk in the garden, and accidentally hit my finger. The cut didn't bleed too much, but it looked purple. My finger was swollen three times its normal size. My daughter wanted to take me to the hospital, but I decided to apply noni juice to my finger. A few minutes later the pain was gone, and three hours later the swelling was down.

I am a busy working mother, involved in community work and singing. I have very little time to rest my body or my voice, so I was having problems projecting my voice. At my last concert I was surprised when my voice came through loud and clear. At first I thought it was because of the acoustics in the building. Then I remembered drinking one ounce of noni juice that morning and another ounce on the way to the concert.

I wish I could convey the benefits of taking noni juice. I am frustrated to see people being ignorant of the help they could receive—some of them waiting to die but not willing to try this alternative.

Complementary Pain Therapies to Noni

There are a number of things you may do to further noni's effectiveness and complement its abilities.

DIETARY/SUPPLEMENTATION CONSIDERATIONS

Increasing the level of the following nutrients in one's diet, or supplementing with these supplements can provide additional firepower in fighting pain:

EPA (eicosapentaenoic acid). A fatty acid that comes from fish such as salmon, tuna, and mackerel, this fatty acid can help normalize the body's inflammation response. It can be effective against inflammatory diseases such as rheumatoid arthritis.

GLA (gamma linolenic acid). This fat is similar to EPA, though its benefits don't seem to be quite as strong as those of EPA. It can be taken in supplement form, usually sold as evening primrose oil. It could be helpful used in combinations with other fatty acids.

ALA (alpha linolenic acid). Found mostly in green vegetables, this is not usually found in supplement form. Great sources of ALA include the chlorophyll-filled "green foods" such as spirulina, wheat grass, alfalfa and chlorella. These foods also contain a number of other very important nutrients, all of which can contribute to the reduction of inflammation and pain.

Turmeric. A spice commonly used in Eastern food dishes, turmeric contains high levels of curcumin, a substance often shown to be as effective as anti-inflammatories like cortisone, ibuprofen and phenylbutazone. Unlike these drugs, however, curcumin is very safe, even when taken in high doses. Studies have shown turmeric (and specifically curcumin) to be effective against rheumatoid arthritis and general joint stiffness and swelling.

Chamomile. This pleasant-tasting herb is an effective anti-inflammatory agent, as well as a mild sedative. It also helps relieve muscle spasms. It has been shown to specifically help with trigeminal neuralgia (facial nerve pain). Chamomile can be used in teas, capsules or compresses.

Cayenne. Also known as capsicum, this red chile pepper provides "warmth" that gives a stimulant to the brain that competes with pain signals. It has been shown to prevent the production of substance-P, a pain-carrying chemical.

DL-phenylalanine. This amino acid form helps fight pain, preventing the breakdown of endorphins. Studies have shown it to be especially effective against chronic pain.7

White willow bark. A very popular herbal, white willow contains salicin, which is converted to salicylic acid, similar to aspirin. It has been used for centuries in various cultures for treating numerous types of aches and pains.

Phosphatidyl serine. This substance aids the nerve cells in conducting impulses, helps the brain to manufacture neurotransmitters and blocks the stress hormone cortisol, which can contribute to an increased perception of pain. It has been shown in a number of studies to improve short-term memory and concentration, which are important in the body's control of pain.

Avoid animal fats. Animal meats, like red meat, pork, and chicken contain fats and other substances that can contribute to symptoms of arthritis, inflammation and general joint pain.

"I rubbed the mixture on my arm and the pain was completely alleviated after only two applications!"

Garrett Bouvier experience relief from a bad wrist after using noni topically.

I was bothered with constant pain in my wrist and forearm for six months following a car accident. I tried chiropractic treatment, physical therapy, and pain medication, but nothing stopped the pain.

When I heard that a noni-based joint support supplement could be used topically, I mixed a few drops with one teaspoon of a noni-based lotion. I rubbed the mixture into my arm and the pain was completely alleviated after only two applications!

OTHER CONSIDERATIONS

As this chapter explains, pain is a complex entity that can accompany other disorders or become its own condition. There are a substantial number of treatments or therapies that may help alleviate pain to discuss here. My suggestion would be to consult one or more of the many excellent reference texts available that adequately outline commonly used and effective anti-pain therapies. Consulting health care providers familiar with these therapies can also be very helpful. With my patients, I found the following anti-pain therapies to be helpful: hypnosis, imagery, total muscle relaxation, abdominal breathing, visualization, distraction, focusing, and mental anesthesia.

Chapter Summary Points

- Chronic pain can result from an underlying ailment (such as arthritis or an injury) and eventually become its own condition.

- Many pain experts believe that pain travels along its own nervous system pathways, which contain gates that open and close. If the gates are closed, the pain can't travel and therefore is minimized. It is believed by many that these gates can begin to malfunction and become "jammed," which allows pain signals to travel continuously and therefore contribute to a condition of chronic pain.

- Chronic pain is one of the most common complaints for which noni has been utilized, both historically and in modern times. Because pain is associated with such a wide variety of ailments, it is one of the most oft-reported symptoms alleviated by noni use.

- Noni is a proven COX 2 enzyme inhibitor, the enzyme responsible for painful inflammation.

- Other of noni's anti-pain properties are terpenes, scopoletin, and its modulation of the brain chemical serotonin.

Chapter
6
Cancer and Noni

When you're young, healthy, and on top of the world, you think your chances of developing cancer are "one in a million." The fact is, every year more than one million Americans find out they have cancer. This equates to a chance of about one in three that you will do one of two things: die of cancer or survive it. This chapter will focus on how to increase your likelihood of survival.

Cancer is scary. It is often thought of as one of the most menacing and deadly of diseases. However, while it can be deadly, modern research has given new hope to cancer patients. Though the number of new cancer cases has not dropped, the success rate for overcoming cancer has seen a slow rise over the years. This means there is a better chance now than ever before that those who have cancer will survive.

More people are surviving cancer due to better and earlier detection methods, more effective diagnostic methods, new drugs, and a better understanding of how the body can naturally fight cancer. One of the most exciting, widely studied natural methods to fight cancer is noni. This chapter will introduce you to some of the cutting edge research that has been done and that is currently underway involving noni and cancer.

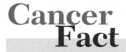

Cancer
Fact

Five-year survival improved significantly for children, from 56 percent in the mid-1970s to 78 percent in the 1990s.

There are different ways people use noni juice to help combat cancer. Some use it for help with cancer prevention, others use it to help supplement a conventional cancer treatment. Some resort to alternative treatment for cancer because conventional methods have not worked and doctors have told them there is "no hope." Another way in which people use noni with their cancer treatment is to use it to help control cancer symptoms or side effects that accompany many cancer treatments. Whatever the reason, noni is proving itself to be a natural power house in the fight against one of our society's most deadliest diseases.

"The cancer was confined within the ovarian capsule and had not spread."

Ann Wilson recounts her harrowing battle with cancer and how she believes noni helped.

I started drinking noni juice more than seven years ago. After hearing many positive stories about the Tahitian people and the science behind noni, I wanted to try it for myself. I started taking two ounces of noni juice twice daily, and in 2000 I upped my dosage to two ounces four times daily—just to feel better.

In June of 2002, at 50 years of age, I began a weight loss program. I lost 36 pounds and so I didn't seem to notice the swelling in my abdomen. On September 14, I started feeling ill, so I made an appointment with my doctor. A sonogram showed a mass on my left ovary the size of a four-month old fetus. On Wednesday, September 18, I had surgery and a cancerous ovarian tumor was found. The doctors performed a full hysterectomy and took biopsies of various organs and lymph nodes for further testing.

After the operation, the surgeon spoke with my husband and family. He explained I probably had a 30 percent chance of living another six months. Ovarian cancer is very deadly, and because its symptoms are hard to detect it spreads easily. He told everyone to put on a happy face and be positive for me as we awaited the lab results.

On Friday the 20th, we received the pathology report, and the results were astounding! The tumor weighed 1032 grams and measured up to 19 centimeters in diameter. But the most amazing discovery was the cancer was confined within the ovarian capsule and had not spread to any surrounding tissue or bodily organs. All the biopsy reports came back negative. This was incredible! The chances of having a cancerous ovarian tumor the size of mine that had not spread to other parts of the body are one in 100,000! It was truly a miracle. If the doctor could have done back flips, I think he would have!

As a precautionary measure, I underwent six treatments of chemotherapy, which ended in January of 2003. I continued to drink noni juice and never experienced the typical nausea that accompanies chemotherapy. I did, however, lose all of my hair and gain 20 pounds.

Having a complete hysterectomy threw me into immediate, full-blown menopause, and I suffered all the typical menopause symptoms from hot flashes to restless sleep. I tried a progesterone cream, but it didn't help. I knew I should be eating soy products for the hormonal balancing effect they have, but every soy product on the market made me want to gag. They taste terrible!

At the same time, Tahitian Noni International introduced the Tahiti Trim® Plan 40. I started using the noni-based progesterone cream as well as the noni-based soy protein drinks (which actually taste good). My hot flashes disappeared along with all of the other symptoms of menopause.

I am thrilled to be alive. After such an ordeal that is what really matters. Today I have a 95 percent chance of survival, and there is no evidence of disease in my body. I truly believe in miracles, and I believe noni juice helped with mine!

Cancer—The No. 2 Killer

Cancer Fact

About 156 people an hour will learn they have cancer this year, according to the American Cancer Society.

Currently, cancer is the leading cause of death in Canada. In the United States, cancer is second only to heart disease as a leading cause of death. Each year, 1.2 million people in the United States are diagnosed with cancer, and each day, 1,700 people in the United States alone die from this disease. This may seem confusing after just reading that your chance to survive cancer has never been higher. The reason cancer continues to be a leading killer is mainly because we live longer, thereby giving more time for diseases such as cancer to develop.

Cancer develops when abnormal cells grow uncontrollably and invade and destroy body tissues. Cancer can occur in almost any organ or tissue in the body. There are ways to fight back, but to understand how to fight back we first need to know how cancer cells develop in the first place.

As cells wear out they replicate themselves. As they divide, cells pass on their genetic information. This genetic code, the DNA, determines what the cell will be and what it will do. One portion of the DNA contains the encoding for a process called "apoptosis." Apoptosis is the time limit of a cell—it contains the information for self-destruction of the cell after it has served its useful purpose. Normal cell growth includes the death of old cells (apoptosis) and the controlled reproduction of new cells. Cancerous cell growth does not include that process.

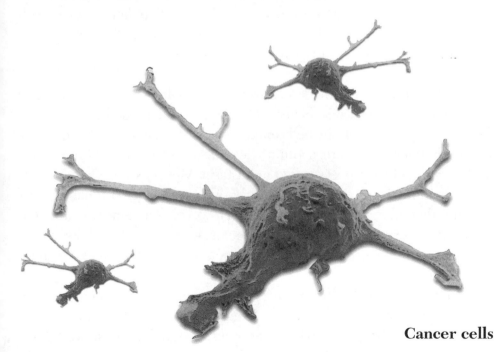

Cancer cells

The Phases of Cancer

There are two phases to cancer. The first phase involves damage to DNA, which can be caused by any number of factors, including carcinogens. The most widely known carcinogens are chemicals. While many carcinogenic chemicals are accidentally introduced to the body, some such as tobacco are self-induced. Other carcinogens include radiation. A 2001 government survey of 3,800 people by the Centers for Disease Control (CDC) and Prevention reported that most Americans carry detectable traces of potentially deadly toxins in their blood and urine. However, when the human body is working properly, these toxins do not turn into cancer. However, when the body's immune system has been compromised, cancer may develop from exposure to toxins.

Of course, genetics is a very powerful determinant of cancer. Some viruses have also been linked to certain cancers. When introduced to the body, carcinogens attack the DNA of the exposed cells. The damage can result in cancer. Not everyone who is exposed to carcinogens contracts cancer; however, the greater the exposure the greater the risk.

The second phase of cancer involves uncontrolled growth. Damaged DNA alone does not cause cancer. However, if a damaged cell does not die or repair itself, then the cell can pass on its damaged DNA sequence. The cycle continues until a tumor develops. Eventually, a tumor may start to spread in a process called metastasis. Metastasis is when cancerous cells move from one part of the body to another. Originally it was thought that metastasis was random. However, current research has shown that certain cancers tend to metastasize to certain body parts. Breast cancer, for instance, often will metastasize to the skeletal system.

Common cancer treatments place a great deal of emphasis on the second phase of uncontrolled growth. If damaged cells can be induced into apoptosis, then the cancer will be stopped or significantly slowed down again. Surgery, radiation, and chemotherapy all try to stop growth. In surgery, the cancerous growth is physically removed. Radiation involves killing cancerous cells by bombarding them with x-rays or gamma rays. Chemotherapy introduces powerful medicines into the body that kill the cancerous cells. Unfortunately, chemotherapy medicines do not differentiate between healthy and sick cells. Most doctors use a combination of these treatments.

Alternative Choices

As research continues, new methods are being tried to help fight cancer. Some of these methods do not focus on the second phase of cancer, but instead focus on boosting the body's immune system that has been compromised in the individual with cancer. These methods are called biological treatments.

In addition, plant extracts used to help fight against cancer have been growing in popularity in the mainstream medical field. Extracts from the red periwinkle—used for leukemia and lymphomas—and etoposide, from the American Mayapple, as well as *Morinda citrifolia* (noni) are just some examples of current plant-based biological therapies. In 2001, at the 92nd Annual Meeting of the American Association for Cancer Research, noni was listed as one of the top ten alternative cancer treatments used in conventional settings.

According to surveys from the American Cancer Society done in 1989, 9 percent of cancer patients at that time were using one or more alternative treatments. Surveys done only ten years later, in 1998, showed that 31 percent of American cancer patients now used alternative therapy. (This number was even higher outside of the United States. In Canada, it was about 42 percent.) This means in ten years the use of alternative methods increased more than three-fold.

Dr. Ralph W. Moss, a well-known cancer researcher, reports there are five main instances when alternative treatment is usually used in the case of cancer. These are:

(1) Primary prevention. People use diet and natural supplements to try and ward off the disease in the first place. Noni itself contains over 150 nutraceuticals important to the body, some of which are known anti-cancer agents.

(2) Secondary prevention. Cancer survivors often use diet and supplements to prevent a recurrence.

(3) Reduction of side effects. During the course of conventional treatment, many patients suffer negative side effects. Some natural products, such as noni, may be used to possibly reduce those side effects.

(4) Modulation of immunity. Many cancers disrupt the immune system. Some people use natural methods of trying to boost the body's immune system in order to ward off disease and to combat the cancer itself. Researcher Dr. Anne Hirazumi Kim has focused much of her published work on this aspect of noni. We'll talk more about her work in a moment.

(5) Treatment of advanced disease. Many patients turn to non-conventional methods once it appears that conventional medicine has nothing further to offer them.

"I Felt 100 Percent Better!"

Stephen had been hospitalized for over three weeks after having surgery for colon cancer. He describes his experience with noni:

The entire time I was in the hospital, my condition was not good. I was completely unable to tolerate any food and had to be fed via an IV. About this time, my sister brought the doctor some information on noni and asked if we could put a few drops under my tongue a couple times a day. The doctor agreed.

So we began the "noni" treatment. About this time, the doctor determined that they would probably need to perform another surgery to check for a blockage in my intestines because I'd had very little movement since the surgery. After only one day of taking the noni, I began to feel some activity in my bowel region. That evening, I had a bowel movement, the first in over three weeks. The next morning my IV was removed and I was started on a liquid diet. One day later I had a "soft" meal and that evening a regular meal. I had regular bowel movements over those few days. The next day I was discharged from the hospital, whereas a few days before I was scheduled for surgery because of my poor response. I felt 100 percent better.

Noni's War on Cancer

Cancer
Preventative

"TAHITIAN NONI® Juice may possess a cancer preventative, and including TAHITIAN NONI® Juice in your diet may help prevent cancer and disease while maintaining overall good health."
—*Annals of the New York Academy of Sciences, Volume 952, at The Conference on Cancer Prevention,"* 10-11-2000.

Cancer is a disease of the cells—all of the more than one hundred known cancers begin with one cell that mutates and eventually leads to wild cell proliferation. One tiny microscopic cell somehow evades the body's defenses and replicates unchecked—one single cell. Noni researcher Dr. Ralph Heinicke believes noni's strongest health benefits is its ability to work at the cellular level, helping abnormally functioning cells (like cancerous cells) to once again regain normal function and to stimulate the body's immune system to fight invading pathogens.

One of the first key studies that involved noni and cancer was presented at the 83rd Annual Meeting of the American Association for Cancer Research in 1992. This study dealt with the anti-tumor activity of noni used on mice suffering from Lewis lung carcinoma.

Anne Hirazumi Kim, Ph.D., considered by many to be one of today's top noni researchers, led a team from the University of Hawaii in a thorough testing of noni and its touted cancer-fighting abilities in cell and animal models. Initially, Dr. Kim's team treated cancerous lung cells with a polysaccharide-rich noni preparation. This did not significantly affect the cancer cells. However, upon introducing peritoneal exudate cells (PEC), model cells for immune function, to the mix of cancerous cells and noni preparation, the PEC defense cells were activated. These cells proceeded to kill a large number of the cancerous cells, ultimately resulting in a significant reduction in tumor growth.

To further test noni's ability to encourage the immunological strengthening response against cancerous cells, the researchers administered different types of noni preparations to mice with Lewis lung cancer, but withheld the noni from a group with cancer. The results of this portion of the study were indeed impressive. The first group, consisting of 78 mice, was given crude noni juice. A second group, considered the control group, was not given noni juice. Of the 55 mice not treated with the juice, not one was cured (or lived longer than 50 days). However, of the 78 mice given the noni juice, 20 mice were cured. Additionally, their survival rates were substantially longer than the untreated mice. In fact, they lived up to 119 percent longer, more than twice as long!

The second experiment, consisting of a control group of 58 and a group of 61 given a noni precipitate (a more concentrated preparation of noni juice), provided similar results. In the control group, not one was cured. However, of the noni-fed group, 20 were cured (which constitutes a 32 percent cure rate). Consequently, and not surprisingly, the survival rates were significantly higher for the noni group—up to 118 percent higher! How did noni produce such an effect in these mice? As pointed out previously, one of the specific goals of this study was to see if noni could stimulate the function of the immune system. Preliminary testing showed that the noni preparation did indeed invigorate the potential anticancer activity of PEC cells, suggesting the strong possibility of noni's ability to strengthen the body's immune system.

In later testing, Dr. Kim and her team conducted a series of studies to determine if noni could enhance the production of macrophages, the cells responsible for literally destroying and consuming dangerous toxins, cells and organisms. They concluded that these tests indicated that noni "could stimulate the activation of macrophages." Specifically, noni stimulated the activity of nitric oxide, tumor necrosis factor-alpha, and interleukin 1ß, all of which are recognized as anticancer agents.

The study also included the testing of noni's action with several well-known anti-cancer agents to see if the therapeutic effects of either the drugs or noni would be enhanced. Dr. Kim concludes that using noni as a supplementary treatment with below-normal doses of anti-cancer drugs such as adriamycin, 5-fluorourcil (5FU) or vincristine could produce excellent benefits with lessened side effects than just the drugs alone.

What do the results of these studies really mean? Basically, Dr. Kim found that components in noni were able to biologically boost the function of the immune system in mice sufficiently so that a significant number of these noni-fed mice survived cancer. While there are certain limitations to this study (mice, not humans, were studied and only one type of cancer was studied), Dr. Kim's research is extremely exciting. The study's conclusion suggests "important clinical applications of noni as a supplemental agent in cancer treatment. . . ."

"He called me his 'miracle man.' "

Robin L. Baggett, a man in the prime of life, tells of his incredible battle with lymphoma.

In September 1997 I noticed a small bump on my neck, but I passed it off as nothing serious. In December of that year my doctor saw the knot on my neck and jumped out of his chair and said, "My God, you have lymphoma!"

Almost the next day I had three doctors working on me and they all said it didn't look good. I was moving forward to start traditional *treatment; however there was a two-week window for me to look at alternatives.*

I took mega doses of TAHITIAN NONI® Juice for the two weeks prior to my first treatment. All the doctors had said my immune system would be terribly impaired by the treatment, and I hoped TAHITIAN NONI® Juice would help boost my immune system. For my treatment, I had 37 radiation treatments on a daily basis. On some days I also had chemo. From the doctors and nurses I heard nothing good about my situation. I was terminally ill. Even with traditional treatment my chances were not good. However, I kept up going to work during the entire treatment.

Over time, I was unable to swallow even water. At that time, I had to stop taking noni juice, and I started going downhill rapidly. One day my wife said, "Why not pour TAHITIAN NONI® Juice in your stomach tube." I took her suggestion. My blood work began improving right away.

There are many ways in which I believe noni improved my situation during my cancer treatment. For example, there is a cream called TAHITIAN NONI® Skin Supplement. I used it on my face and neck to prevent the customary burning and blistering of the skin. Even the technicians that helped me get onto the radiation table every day noticed that my skin was not being affected like all their other patients.

"I completed my traditional treatment in March 1998. My next appointment with my doctor was the first time I ever saw him smile. He came in the office with his thumbs in the air and said that all signs of the cancer appear to have gone. He called me his "miracle man!"

Dr. Mian-Ying Wang

A study by another top-notch cancer expert also supports the notion that noni can aid the body in fighting cancer. This study, conducted by Dr. Mian-Ying Wang and other researchers at the University of Illinois College of Medicine at Rockford, showed that a group of mice given a mixture of water and noni juice had better cancer prevention ability than water-fed mice. The study fed one group of mice a solution consisting of 10 percent noni juice for one week. The control group was only fed water. On the last day of the experiment, each animal in both groups was given a specific dose of DMBA, a known cancer-causing agent.

Twenty-four hours after administering the DMBA, the vital organs—the heart, liver, lung and kidneys—of the animals were examined and tested using a DNA isolation process. Here's what the examination revealed.

Markers used to determine the cancer activity of a substance are called DNA adduct markers. The lower the number, the more protection one has against developing cancer. The group given noni was examined and then compared against the group not given noni. In the group given noni, the quantity of these markers found in the liver were reduced by 60 percent. In the heart, they were reduced by 75 percent. There was a 70 percent reduction in the lungs and a 90 percent reduction in the kidneys. Again, these results are very exciting. (See Figure 1.)

Figure 1

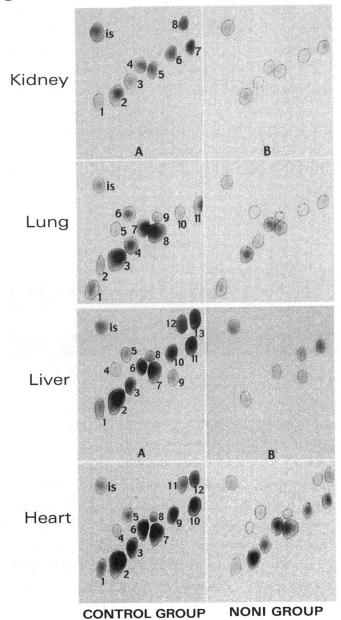

CONTROL GROUP   NONI GROUP

Radiographic Density Pattern of DNA adduct markers (single nucleotide) from two-dimensional thin chromatography. *In simple terms, the markers on the right, which are taken from the group given noni juice and which show less density, indicate more protection against cancer.*

Dr. Wang has continued her experiments with noni and cancer and in 2001 she published her study results in the *Annals of the New York Academy of Sciences*. A summary of another study with rats completed by Dr. Wang and her associates is shown in Table 1. This study addressed the hypothesis that TAHITIAN NONI® Juice possesses a cancer preventative effect at the initiation stage of carcinogenesis. Preliminary data suggest that pretreatment for one week with TAHITIAN NONI® Juice in drinking water at a concentration of 10% was able to reduce DMBA-DNA adduct formation (marker for developing cancer) in rats.

Table 1.

Pretreatment with rats drinking 10% TAHITIAN NONI® Juice

% Cancer Reduction (Males)		% Cancer Reduction (Females)
Heart	60%	30%
Lungs	50%	41%
Liver	70%	42%
Kidney	90%	80%

Dr. Wang's studies in rats suggest that TAHITIAN NONI® Juice may prevent cancer at its initiation stage by blocking or decreasing carcinogen induced DNA adduct formation. In addition, she believes TAHITIAN NONI® Juice has other cancer-preventing qualities as well. She has shown in vitro (test tube) and in vivo (body) that TAHITIAN NONI® Juice reduces cancer growth through its scavenging reactive oxidative species (ROS), its quenching lipid peroxides (LPO), and its anti-inflammatory effect.

Studies have shown that eating fruits and vegetables may reduce free radical damage and lipid peroxidation in cigarette smokers, resulting in fewer cancer risks. Some fruits and vegetable are sources of antioxidants, including noni. Interestingly, studies from the New York Apple Research Development show that isolating out a single compound in fruits (such as vitamin C) is not nearly as effective as eating the fruit just as mother nature intended. Their studies show that just 100 grams of fresh apple with skin had the same anti-cancer properties of 1,500 milligrams of vitamin C. It is the plant's combination of flavonoids and polyphenols that is so important in health. This goes against what many have believed. For years people have assumed it was better to stock up on vitamins and minerals isolated from substances and sold as a pill in bottle. Research now shows it is better to go back to whole foods.

In an effort to see if the antioxidants, flavonoids, and polyphenols in noni could help protect individuals from cigarette smoke by scavenging oxygen free radicals and quenching lipid peroxides, Dr. Wang recently conducted another study.

This study was a one-month double blinded, randomized, placebo-controlled clinical trial. It was designed to test the protective effect of noni on plasma SAR and LPO in current smokers. The smokers were daily supplied with two ounces of noni juice or a placebo twice a day for 30 days. The plasma SAR and LPO levels were determined before and after the trial by TBN and LPO assay, respectively. The LPO and SAR concentration in the noni-fed group showed a 23 percent reduction of LPO and a 27 percent reduction of SAR. The LPO and SAR levels in the placebo group remained the same. Dr. Wang is now continuing this line of research with an even larger number of participants.

Other Researchers

In another study done in the 1990s, scientists in Japan published an article in *Cancer Letters* that again validated the theory that *Morinda citrifolia* shows cancer-fighting abilities. In this study, the scientists injected *ras* cells (cells that are precursors to many malignant growths) with a substance called damnacanthal, which they obtained from noni. They observed that the injection of damnacanthal significantly inhibited the *ras* cells from reproducing.

Currently, researchers at the University of Hawaii are doing a study that involves noni and humans. During this study, Dr. Brian Issell is monitoring the CAT scans of cancer patients who use noni to see if there are any significant changes in the scans. In addition, the researchers are analyzing blood and urine samples from participants to check for toxicity and safety issues. Phase I of the study has shown "positive results." "So far, we have discovered that there really are chemicals in noni that slow down the growth of certain tumor cells," reports Dr. Issell. To do the study, Dr. Issell was awarded $340,000 by the National Institutes of Health, which in and of itself is an indication of how interested the medical community is in noni juice.

Cox 2 Enzyme

There is an interesting link between the COX 2 enzyme, cancer, and noni. In chapter five we talked about Dr. John R. Vane who discovered the COX enzyme that converted body acids into prostaglandins that can cause inflammation around joints. This discovery led to extensive research on the COX enzyme and its relationship to arthritis. It also led to a later discovery (in 1991) by Dr. Daniel L. Simmons. He discovered there are really two COX enzymes, COX 1 and COX 2. Dr. Simmons is an oncologist, and he found the COX 2 enzyme while studying cancer. It was only later the major link between COX 2 and arthritis was made. The current COX 2 prescription inhibitors are also prescribed for several different types of genetic cancer.

For example, COX 2 frequently shows up in a common form of stomach cancer. In addition, cancerous tumors in the colon, pancreas, breast, lung, liver and prostate all have increased amounts of COX 2. In the July 2001 issue of *Clinical Cancer Research*, Finnish scientists reported that they examined tumors from 43 patients with a type of stomach cancer that resembles colon cancer. Of these 43 patients, 25 showed evidence of the increased COX 2 enzyme. Some researchers believe that a new critical avenue to study may be how to combat cancer using COX 2 inhibition. Remember, TAHITIAN NONI® Juice is a proven natural COX 2 inhibitor.

Noni's Front Line

In the last section we talked about studies that confirm noni is a powerful natural supplement in the fight against cancer. In this section, let's briefly cover some of noni's top fighters—the ingredients in noni that make it so effective. There are at least five specific substances found in noni that have anti-cancer properties.

- **Anthraquinones.** The anthraquinones in noni help fight inflammation, bacteria, parasites, and tumors. Anthraquinones are also used to boost the body's immune system. Damnacanthal, an anthraquinone found in noni, inhibits the formation of tumors by interfering with the growth of ras cells. It is believed that other anthraquinones, such as alizarin that is also in noni, cut off the blood supply to tumors, depriving them of their nutrients. This can slow the growth of tumors.

- **Epigallocatechin gallate (EGCg)**—EGCg is a polyphenolic flavonoid antioxidant that is found in abundance in noni. Researchers from Purdue University reported EGCg was extremely successful at killing tumor cells by interfering with tNOX (the tumor-associated activity of NOX) but not with normal NOX. EGCg has also been shown to limit the activity of breast cancer tumor cells grown in the laboratory, but not normal healthy breast cells.

- **Monoterpenes**—Monoterpenes have been shown to prevent cancer at both the beginning and progression stages by inducing cellular apostosis (or cellular death). Monoterpenes show no toxic effects on the body even in large quantities. One of the most common monoterpenes scientists have examined is limonene (found in lemons and in noni juice). The monoterpene limonene has been shown to help prevent mammary, liver, lung, and other cancers. It has been used to treat a variety of rodent cancers, including breast and pancreatic carcinomas. In addition, in vitro data suggest it may be effective in treating some forms of leukemia. One particular study showed that limonene was a major factor in specifically resisting breast cancer. Some researchers declared limonene and limonene-related monoterpenes should be considered as "a new class of therapeutic agents for treating breast cancer."

- **Polysaccharides**—Polysaccharides help block mutated cells from attaching to healthy cells, such as in metastasis. In one study done at the Medical Research Institute in Tokyo, Japan, researchers injected rats with colonic carcinogens. Four weeks after the cancerous injection, researchers began injecting the mice three times a week for eight weeks with polysaccharides. They found that the polysaccharide-treated rats had 44 percent fewer colonic tumors than the control rats and their survival rate increased 150 percent.

- **Terpenoid compounds**—The specific terpenes in noni are eugenol, beta-carotene, and ursolic acid. Eugenol is an active germicide as well as a smooth-muscle relaxer. It has been involved with various studies on breast cancer. Beta-carotene is associated with reducing cancers of the lung, skin, cervix, prostate, and respiratory and gastrointestinal tracts. Beta-carotene is believed to function by boosting the thymus gland that distributes T cells. Beta-carotene should be used in moderate amounts. Ursolic acid has positive effects on treating cancer both externally and internally. It has been found to be effective as both an anti-inflammatory and as an anti-tumor agent.

Boosting Anti-Cancer Defenses in the Body

In addition to containing ingredients that have been linked to anti-cancer properties, Dr. Kim's research has shown noni may modulate the production, activity, and effectiveness of some immune system agents, most of which are directly responsible for warding off diseases such as cancer. These immune system agents are nitric oxide, interleukins, interferon, tumor necrosis factor, lipopolysaccharide, and natural killer cells.

Nitric Oxide
The benefits of nitric oxide are being loudly touted in the medical world today. One of nitric oxide's abilities is to ward off cancer attacks on the cells. In her published work, Dr. Kim states, "Nitric oxide produced by activated macrophages plays a role in the host protection against pathogens as well as tumors." She also states that nitric oxide can kill pathogens by destroying the DNA synthesis of such cells and by poisoning them.

Interleukins
Another immune system agent that noni may modulate is interleukins. Interleukins are hormones that carry messages from one immune cell to

another, informing the receiving cell to speed up its multiplication when in danger of invading pathogens. There are several different types of interleukins, and they are usually classified by numbers, such as inter-leukin-2. Interleukin-2 is closely tied to the body's anti-cancer mechanisms. Interleukins also enhance the production of B-cell antibodies, and promote the cytotoxicity of Natural killer (NK) cells. They also can play a role in activating T-lymphocytes.

Interferon

Interferons are another component of the body's immune system. As with interleukins, there are several types of interferons. The type of interferon that noni is believed to modulate is interferon-y. Interferon-y was originally thought to be anti-viral. More and more, it also shows up in the body during the immune system's fight against cancer. It is believed that it helps in the activation of macrophages and the overall process of cell-mediated immunity. Dr. Kim's research also makes mention of interferons in connection to noni and its immune-boosting properties.

Tumor Necrosis Factor

Tumor necrosis factor (TNF) is a substance secreted by various macrophages (which may be modulated by noni) to kill tumors. It is believed the tumor necrosis factor plays a principal role in the immune system's fight against cancer.

Lipopolysaccharide (LPS)

Certain bacteria have an outer layer that is composed mainly of lipopolysaccharide. Consequently, the presence of LPS in the blood stream usually means a bacterial infection. The immune system reacts to the presence of LPS and tries to eliminate the assumed invading organism. If LPS is able to get into the bloodstream in ways other than through bacteria, (such as by ingesting noni which may modulate LPS production) the body may increase its immune system activity.

Natural Killer Cells (NK)

Noni is believed to modulate another vital component of the body's immune system— natural killer cells. These cells are considered deadly to many invaders. The NK cells can recognize and destroy virally infected cells, as well as some tumor cells.

"The Cancer Was In Complete Remission"

Angela, 49 years old, provides the details of her fantastic recovery from a near-fatal bout with brain cancer.

In April 1997 I lost the use of the left side of my body. The doctors couldn't figure out what was wrong so they put a soft boot on my left leg up to my knee so that I could walk. A few weeks later after a sauna at the gym, I had a seizure. I was taken to the hospital and x-rays showed that I had a brain tumor, which had caused my brain to swell. They said it was an anaplastic oligodendroglioma, which is a very rare type of cancer with an extremely low survival rate. Immediately a neurosurgeon operated on me, but he could not remove the entire tumor without affecting vitally functioning parts of my brain. I was then given six weeks of radiation and one year of chemotherapy.

Not surprisingly, the chemotherapy made me deathly ill with weakness, nausea, vomiting, and fever. I lost 35 pounds. During the next few months, I was in and out of the hospital and was too weak to participate in any of my normal activities. I had to take early retirement from work and was put on permanent long-term disability. My oncologist told me that I was terminal, that there was no hope. Despite this, I firmly decided that I was going to live.

A short time later, I started taking about eight ounces of noni juice a day on the advice of a friend. After calling the office of a nutritionist familiar with using noni for cancer, I increased my consumption to a full bottle a day for the next four weeks. Next I went to Texas to consult with a nutritionist and homeopathic practitioner. His tests indicated that I had the body of a 73-year-old, though I was 48. Based on the results of his tests he added various supplements and advised me to continue drinking eight ounces of noni juice daily.

Several days into my treatment, I noticed my strength returning and I started to gain weight. I spent the next year working on healing myself. I used meditation, visualization, hands-on healing, and motivational tapes and books. I modified my diet to include more fruits and vegetables and tried to eliminate pesticides and preservatives by eating organic foods. As I gained strength I started an organic garden, revamped my backyard, joined a bowling league, and took golf lessons. For about eight months, I drank about eight ounces of noni juice daily. In April 1999, my doctors told me the cancer was in complete remission.

Complementary Therapies to Noni

GENERAL LIFE STYLE RECOMMENDATIONS

Nutritional choices. Choose a diet that is predominantly plant-based, rich in a variety of vegetables and fruits, legumes, seeds, whole grains and foods that have been minimally processed.

Body weight. Avoid being overweight or significantly underweight (the latter being mostly a problem with elderly individuals).

Physical activity. The point is this—be active. If all of the benefits of exercise could be combined in a pill form (and I'm sure there are pills marketed as such), people would flock to this "miracle" pill. If your occupational activity is low or moderate, take an hour's break to engage in a brisk walk or something of similar intensity each day. In addition, try to engage in vigorous physical activity (where you actually sweat) for a total of at least an hour each week.

Pinpointing the effects of fitness on cancer risk is not easy because people who are physically fit tend to have healthier lifestyles overall. In several studies, scientists have observed that people who live sedentary lifestyles have a higher risk of developing different types of cancer than their more active counterparts. Confirming these findings, a study carried out at the Harvard School of Public Health found that women who participated in college athletics had a 35 percent lower rate of breast cancer and a 60 percent lower rate of cancers in the reproductive system in later years than those who had not been involved in athletics.

DIET/NUTRITION RECOMMENDATIONS

It is no secret that diet is extremely important to enjoying good health. But most of us know that today's prevalent lifestyles often make it difficult to consume an ideal diet. Thus dietary supplements—like noni—can make substantial contributions to the fulfilling of certain nutritional needs that our bodies may have.

But noni is not alone in its nutritional value. There are many things we can do to improve our dietary habits and make full use of the nutrition possibilities available to most of us. The majority of those familiar with noni would agree that noni's healthful benefits are probably enhanced by the presence of other necessary nutrients. The following should be considered in not only improving your dietary habits, but also as a way to improve noni's health-promoting action.

Fruits and vegetables. Eat 15–30 ounces (one to two pounds, or five servings) of a variety of fruits and vegetables daily all year long. If that seems like a lot, it really isn't. Fruits and vegetables are mostly water, and water is heavy. For instance, a good size pear or apple can weigh in the neighborhood of half a pound, so only two similar servings of fruit, combined with two or three servings of vegetables, puts you where you want to be. Though we haven't discussed this much, there is considerable evidence that sprouts and grasses, such as wheat grass and bean sprouts, are not only nutrient rich but also high in anti-cancer compounds.

If you're wondering what types of fruits/vegetables to eat, variety is the key. But it is also very important to eat more vegetables than fruit (about a 65–35 percent ratio), with leafy, green vegetables comprising the significant portion of your vegetable intake.

Other plant foods. Eat approximately seven daily servings of a variety of the following "energy" foods: 1) cereals (but avoiding those that are highly processed), 2) legumes and peas, and 3) roots and tubers.

Alcohol. This is a drug, and an addictive one at that, which interferes with the metabolism of many nutrients. It is a potent carcinogen and a promoter of poor dietary habits. While some research indicates that red wine (which may contain cancer-fighting ingredients) could be beneficial, the risks associated with excess alcohol consumption far outweigh its potential benefits. In fact, some research suggests that women with any degree of breast cancer risk should avoid alcohol entirely.

Meat (domesticated red meat, beef, pork, and lamb). The available evidence suggests that it is best to consume very little red meat. You can obtain most of the necessary nutrients that red meat provides, such as protein and iron, from other sources. If you must eat red meat, go for the leanest cut possible. Great alternatives to red meat include fish, vegetable products like legumes and soy, skinless poultry, and game animals or birds.

Fats and oils. Limit consumption of fatty foods, particularly those of animal origin. Choose modest amounts of vegetable oils. These should be mostly polyunsaturated oils, like sunflower or soy oils, or monounsaturated oils, such as olive oil.

Salt. Try to limit consumption of salted foods and the use of extra table salt. Using herbs and spices can do wonders for adding flavor.

Preparation of food. Avoid eating charred meats. Foods that are cooked by steaming, boiling, poaching, stewing, or baking should be the preferred methods of preparation.

Tobacco. This one is simple: Avoid it entirely.

SUPPLEMENTATION

There are a host of substances—herbs, vitamins, minerals, phytohormones all fit into this category—that have anti-cancer benefits. Some work to prevent cancer, while others are adept at helping the cancer sufferer regain energy and experience a minimizing of symptoms. While there is no way we could adequately discuss here the benefits of all supplements that have cancer-fighting benefits, the following is a list of the substances most recognized for their anti-cancer capabilities.

Vitamin C with bioflavonoids. While many vitamins and minerals can help fight cancer, vitamin C has been shown time and time again to be a powerful antioxidant as well as a cancer fighting agent (especially when coupled with bioflavonoids). Research has shown that vitamin C plays a role in fighting cancer of the breast, stomach, pancreas, rectum, cervix, esophagus and lungs.

Soy isoflavones. Also called phytoestrogens, isoflavones have the ability to block the carcinogenic effects of estrogen in breast tissue. They also inhibit activity by the enzymes that promote cancer cell growth, and can interfere with the blood vessel network necessary for a tumor to survive. Compounds found in isoflavones resemble closely the drug tamoxifen, which is used to fight breast cancer.

Indole-3 carbinol. Found in cruciferous vegetables like broccoli and cabbage, these compounds have been linked to the prevention of both breast and prostate cancers.

Essential fatty acids. Though there is still research to be carried out, there is plenty of data to suggest that essential fatty acids can inhibit the growth of existing cancers and lower the risk of certain cancers.

Vitamins A and E. Both of these essential vitamins have been shown time and again to aid the body's immune systems. They can help repair tissue damaged by radiation or chemotherapy, diminish the effects of such treatments and slow the development of various types of cancer.

B-complex vitamins. There is ample research indicating that many B vitamins have a prominent role in helping the body perform the necessary functions to rid itself of cancerous cells. Vitamin B12 has been shown to help battle lung cancer, and a deficiency of vitamin B6 has been linked to the creation of certain malignant tumors.

Pau d'Arco. Very popular as a cancer fighter, there is ample evidence to show that it may indeed fight cancer and, specifically, reverse tumor growth.

Other supplements. The list could go on and on, but here are a few more worth investigating—coenzyme Q10, acidophilus, amino acids, germanium, selenium, vitamin D, spirulina/chlorella, ginseng, barberry root, calcium/magnesium combination, lycopene, shark liver oil, cat's claw, maitake, shitake and reishi mushrooms, d-glucaric acid, kelp, and garlic.

MISCELLANEOUS COMPLEMENTARY THERAPIES TO NONI

Seek emotional and psychological support. The will to live and be happy is paramount. There is ample evidence linking the emotional state of body and mind with the development of cancer.

Join a support group. This coincides with the above suggestion, but studies indicate that becoming involved in such a group is linked with significantly longer survival times.

Practice stress-reduction techniques. Exercise therapies involving stress reduction, such as yoga, can also play a pivotal role in the positive response to cancer.

Laugh every day. Laughter certainly is the "best" medicine.

Consider a detoxification program. Detoxification programs, which include a liver "flush" or juice fast, can aid the body in helping direct its energy towards the most menacing toxin: cancer.

Improve spirituality. Spiritual health is also important to maintaining good health. Though difficult to pin scientific explanations on how it helps, studies have made definite links with religious conviction, or a strong belief system, and the successful treatment of cancer and other diseases.

Chapter Summary Points

- Cancer continues to be this nation's number two killer even though more cases of cancer are being cured each year.

- Despite recent advancements in cancer treatment, noni offers a viable and supporting therapy to help fight cancer and lessen side effects of other treatments, such as chemotherapy.

- Research by Dr. Anne Hirazumi Kim, Dr. Main-Ying, Dr. Brian Issell, and others have given real, scientific proof to noni's effectiveness in relation to some cancers.

- There are at least five known anti-cancer substances in noni. These are: terpenoid compounds, polysaccharides, monoterpenes, Epigallocatechin gallate, anthraquinones.

- The body has various immune cells and substances, such as interferon, nitric oxide, and natural killer cells that effectively seek and destroy cancerous cells. Noni may help modulate these substances and in turn created a stronger immune system.

- There are tremendous amounts of data indicating that rigorous attention to diet, dietary supplements, exercise, stress-release therapies and other therapies can have a profoundly positive impact on cancer. I also believe that if incorporated into a lifestyle of healthful habits, noni can be of great benefit for the cancer patient.

Chapter
7
Chronic Disease

It seems there are as many different definitions of chronic disease as there are different chronic diseases. Let me give you some examples.

Some experts call chronic disease a medical problem that is permanent, disabling, nonreversible, and expected to require a long period of supervision or care. This sounds like a good definition until you consider that most doctors consider obesity a chronic disease. Obesity is not permanent or nonreversible. So that leads us to a new definition.

A second common definition of chronic disease is a condition whose symptoms may be ameliorated with treatment but the underlying condition cannot be cured. This is a little closer to the truth; however, I have seen chronic cases during my practice where the underlying condition has been cured through proper care and a well-rounded treatment plan.

A third common definition for chronic disease is a medical problem that will not improve, lasts a lifetime, or recurs. Again, I have concerns with this definition.

While chronic disease is never easy, it is not a "death sentence." A definition for chronic disease that I think most of us can agree on is, "a disease that has a long course of illness." Chronic illness usually doesn't get better "spontaneously," but it may respond positively to extended treatment, both conventional and alternative.

The Many Faces
of Chronic Disease

AIDS	Chronic Fatigue	Heart Disease
Arthritis	Diabetes	Obesity
Asthma	Epilepsy	Stroke
Cancer	Fibromyalgia	

Researchers say seven out of 10 deaths are the result of chronic illness. Heart disease, cancer, and diabetes are considered to be chronic, and they are the big killers in America and in other parts of the world. Each of these "big three" is the main topic for other chapters of this book. Therefore, I am going to focus this chapter on chronic illness that isn't one of the "big killers," but which is still disabling.

In talking about chronic illness, my main, underlying point is that these are NOT nonreversible conditions as some think. Both past and current experience as a medical professional has taught me that individuals from all walks of life have overcome or have effectively managed many of the illnesses that we classify as chronic disease.

Health
Fact

Approximately one in 544 people in the United States has CFIDS. That adds up to more than 500,000.

Chronic Fatigue

Few death certificates list chronic fatigue as a "cause of death," but this illness certainly can be the cause of many problems during a person's lifetime. That said, chronic fatigue is a chronic illness for which many find relief through naturals means such as noni juice.

To be clinically diagnosed with chronic fatigue, (technically known as chronic fatigue and immune dysfunction syndrome or CFIDS), a person must have severe fatigue for six months or more, and have other "related" symptoms such as substantial impairment in short-term memory or concentration, sore throat, tender lymph nodes, muscle pain, multi-joint pain without swelling or redness, headaches, or unrefreshing sleep.

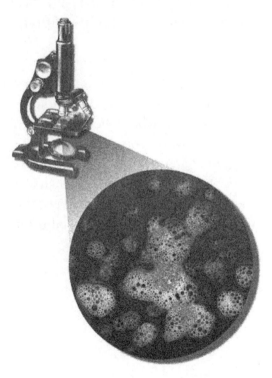

Infection is one of the leading causes of Fatigue

The majority of people with chronic fatigue are women from their teens to late seventies. Many with chronic fatigue remember a "trigger" event that seemed to mark the onset of their condition. Often times persons seeking relief from symptoms of CFIDS feel stigmatized when doctors attribute their symptoms to psychological causes. For that reason, 39 percent of patients with bona fide CFIDS were secretive about their symptoms in some circumstances.

After all, years ago when patients told their doctors of having muscle aches, overwhelming fatigue, depression, headaches, decreased mental abilities, and sleeplessness they were sent home with few or no answers. The good news is that it does not have to be this way! There is now more knowledge than ever as to its causes and how to manage it. You can live actively with CFIDS, especially if a holistic health plan of diet, exercise, supplementation—including noni—and other lifestyle changes is actively employed.

Take for instance Steven Hall, M.D., a cranio-sacral therapist. Dr. Hall reported to me that one of his patients, a 55-year-old female had lived fifteen years with chronic fatigue when she finally came to see him and experienced a complete recovery from her syndrome. Three years later, however, she once again began experiencing CFIDS symptoms after suffering from a viral infection. Dr. Hall reported that after incorporating noni into her daily health regime for only five days, the patient improved by about 90 percent, and she was again in virtual remission.

"My hair became more lustrous, and my optimism returned."

Laura Davis, a 16-year-old teenager from Canada uses noni juice to balance the effects of an under-active thyroid.

I experienced symptoms of an under-active thyroid for about one year before I was diagnosed with hypothyroidism. I started taking four ounces of noni juice every morning. In less than a week my energy level increased and the swelling in my neck went down considerably. My hair become more lustrous and my optimism returned.

Currently I am taking one and a half ounces of noni juice every evening before I go to bed. When I take the noni juice at night I have a much better sleep and feel wide awake in the morning. When I forget to take my noni juice I soon feel the effects of low hormones. I enjoy my life much more when I take noni juice regularly.

Noni and Energy

One of the most common complaints from those who suffer from CFIDS is that they have no energy. Energy plays a crucial role in every process involved in keeping the human body alive. Without energy there is no growth and no cell replication—without energy there can also be no life. So a key to optimal health is what is generally known as energy balance.

For human beings, the negotiable currency of energy comes mainly in the forms of glucose and triglycerides. These we calculate in calories, which are a measure of heat. Each of us must burn a certain number of calories in order to maintain our basal metabolic rate, or BMR, which are those necessary functions of breathing, circulation, digestion, and so on that keep us alive. And so that means we must burn, and thus have stored or consumed, a minimum number of calories per day.

If calories were all we needed—the way a car needs only gasoline—the dietary considerations of life would indeed be easy. But even a car needs more than gasoline—otherwise there would be no need for mechanics. Just like a car, our bodies need a certain level of preventative maintenance. Your physician can help you with some of this maintenance, and you'll do some of it consciously (like brushing your teeth, exercising, and choosing your foods wisely). But most of it your body accomplishes on its own, provided you keep it supplied with the materials to do so. In this regard, physical activity and nutrition are the primary tools your body needs to keep up these functions.

Energy, like many things in life, needs to be in balance in order for bodily systems to work properly. Overfill your gas tank or put in too much oil, and you not only have a mess, but you can also seriously damage your car. When we eat, our bodies take the basic elements of food—the macronutrients of protein, carbohydrate, fat, and others—and transform them into forms of fuel our bodies can use. That fuel is then converted into energy by the cells. Metabolism consists on one level of the processing of raw energy (eating, digestion, combustion, and exhaust) and on another level, of cellular "housekeeping." And it requires more than just calories to keep these interlocking and intertwined systems working—otherwise we could just eat candy bars all day.

So what does noni have to do with the body's effective management of energy? If the body is to operate at an optimal level, every cell must function optimally, which means a proper consumption and conversion of energy. However, we all know that our bodies generally operate in a less than optimum manner, thereby deteriorating or skewing the balance of energy. As we've already discussed, noni, and specifically many of its compounds, can provide individual cells with the needed nutrients to allow "sick" or malfunctioning cells to repair themselves and perform at peak level. It is my belief, as well as that of many others, that noni can positively affect the basic function, including the metabolism and utilization of each cell in the body, thereby bringing about peak performance. One only has to hear the feedback of thousands of noni users concerning the effect of noni on energy levels. Most of these people probably consume more calories than they utilize, yet they feel that they have very little energy to perform the day's tasks. After using noni, even for a short time, the majority report a significant improvement in their moods, "pep," and the energy to achieve what they want. In essence, noni seems to enhance the body's utilization of energy.

Fibromyalgia

Who doesn't occasionally feel sore, achy, or stiff after a weekend of sports activities or heavy gardening? We all do. For those people with fibromyalgia, however, achy, stiff feelings are constant—lasting for months and years—and they are much more severe than normal soreness. In the next few paragraphs, let's talk about some of the symptoms commonly reported from those with fibromyalgia, and then let's talk about how noni can help.

Health
Fact

The prevalence of fibromyalgia is higher in women (3.4 percent) than in men (0.5 percent). Women's symptoms are also more severe than men's are.

Intense pain. Pain is the most common complaint associated with fibromyalgia, affecting about 97 percent of patients. Unlike the pain of bursitis, osteoarthritis, or tendonitis, which is usually relegated to a specific joint or area, this pain can be felt over the entire body and is "deep," sharp, dull, throbbing or aching. The pain is also usually felt in the muscles and connective tissues, rather than in the joints, though joint pain in fibromyalgia sufferers is also fairly common.

The pain can come on gradually with no apparent trigger, or can come on suddenly with or without a triggering factor, such as housework or exercise. And it can become so intense that even prescription pain-killers won't do much to stem it. Many patients also tell of incredibly intense headaches with accompanying pain in the neck and shoulders.

Extreme fatigue. Next to the pain and overall soreness/tenderness, fatigue is the most common complaint linked with fibromyalgia. We all know what it feels like to be tired. But feeling constantly fatigued is another matter. Fibromyalgia causes a constant fatigue that limits the sufferer in her activities, whether it is work, gardening or even light house work. This fatigue can make patients say that they consistently feel tired even when they have had plenty of sleep and should feel rested. Some patients admit to feeling sleepy, though the more common complaint is that of general exhaustion without feeling drowsy or sleepy. This could be compared to having the flu or the feeling after long mental exertion.

Depression. Depression is also a key symptom in fibromyalgia patients. In fact, anxiety and depression severe enough to interfere with daily activities occur in at least half of all sufferers.

Morning stiffness. More than three quarters of fibromyalgia sufferers feel severe stiffness in the morning upon arising. This stiffness creates a feeling of the need to loosen before beginning the day's activities. The stiffness can be extensive, spreading from the muscles and joints of the back, arms and legs.

"Trigger" points. Many patients suffer sharp, throbbing pain that is usually accompanied by what we refer to as "trigger points," localized areas of tenderness usually around joints (though not the joints themselves) that hurt when pressed, as with a finger. These are not areas of deep pain, but rather superficial areas seemingly under the surface of the skin, such as over the elbow or shoulder.

Chronic headaches. More than half of all fibromyalgia sufferers suffer from chronic headaches. They are often caused by tightness in and contraction of the muscles of the neck and head, and are usually referred to as "tension" headaches or "muscle-contraction" headaches.

Irritable bowel syndrome. A condition characterized by abdominal cramps and pain and periods of alternating diarrhea and constipation, irritable bowel syndrome (IBS) is found in about one-third of all fibromyalgia patients.

Overwhelming fatigue. Most people with CFIDS are fatigued most of the time. Occasionally, they have periods—that is short spans of time lasting for several hours or days during which they feel better.

Frequent infections. Many CFIDS patients have recurrent sinus or respiratory infections, sore throats, swollen glands, bladder infections or vaginal, bowel, or skin yeast infections. Some have a recurrent red bumpy rash that is resistant to treatment. They often find that this rash goes away for the first time in years when they have their bowel fungal overgrowth treated. Abdominal gas, cramps, and bloating are also very common, as is alternating diarrhea and constipation. These digestive complaints are attributed to spastic colon and are often triggered by bowel yeast or parasitic infections. Poor food absorption and food sensitivities may also play a significant role in the onset of bowel symptoms.

Brain fog. A condition characterized by cloudy thinking and mental lethargy, "brain fog" is almost routine. Chronic fatigue patients often suffer from poor memory and occasionally from confusion. Brain fog is one of the most frustrating symptoms of CFIDS for some patients and is often the scariest.

Achiness. Chronic diffuse achiness in both muscles and joints is also very common in chronic fatigue patients. For most, this achiness is part of their fibromyalgia.

Increased thirst. When I would meet a new patient who had a water bottle in hand, I would usually know what the main complaint would be. As part of their hormonal problems, people with chronic fatigue have increased urine output and therefore increased thirst. A classic description of these patients is that they "drink like a fish and pee like a race horse." Drinking a lot of water is very important. In fact many CFIDS patients find that they need to drink two to three times as much liquid as the average person.

Allergies. Fatigue patients often have a history of being sensitive to many foods and medications. They often get away with small doses of medications and respond adversely to normal or large doses. Fortunately, severe environmental sensitivity is much less common. I find that food and other sensitivities usually improve when the adrenal insufficiency and yeast or parasitic overgrowth are treated.

There is probably no one single cause of fibromyalgia. Rather, it seems most patients may have several contributing factors that comprise the cause of their particular condition. Moreover, these factors vary widely from patient to patient. In one it may be an emotional trauma, coupled with a bout of depression. In another, it may be one or more serious bouts of flu that mark the onset of fibromyalgia. In this sense, fibromyalgia is still a sort of "mystery" condition. On the same line of thinking, since fibromyalgia may be caused by multiple factors, it is best treated with programs centered on the whole person—the physical, emotional, mental and spiritual. Many such programs utilize dietary supplements such as magnesium, antioxidants, calcium—and noni—to either lessen symptoms or completely reverse the condition.

Noni and Pain

As you can see, one of the biggest complaints of those with fibromyalgia is the constant feeling of stiffness, soreness, and pain. One of pain's biggest culprits is an enzyme called the COX 2 enzyme. In chapter five, we talked about this enzyme and how noni has been proven to slow down the body's production of it. However, let's do a quick review. Most pain is the result of the COX 2 enzyme burning up Arachidonic acid that turns into prostaglandins, which fuel inflammation and pain. If you slow down the production of COX 2, you slow down the body's ability to feel pain and experience inflammation. For years people have relied on non-steroidal anti-inflammatories (NSAIDs) to stop pain. These drugs can cause gastric ulcers, upper GI bleeding, and colitis in many people. The reason for this is because NSAIDS not only slow down the production of COX 2, but they also slow down the production of COX 1, which is an enzyme used in the body to protect the stomach lining.

In the last decade, a lot of research has been conducted on finding a product that would slow down or stop COX 2, but leave COX 1 alone. A few years ago, Tahitian Noni International decided to study the effects noni had on COX 1 and COX 2. Dr. Chen Shu, Jarakae Jensen, and others at the Tahitian Noni International research laboratory proved that TAHITIAN NONI® Juice was a selective inhibitor of COX 2. In addition, the juice did very little, if any damage to the COX 1 enzyme. In other words, this natural juice from French Polynesia is a natural pain killer without side effects!

Asthma

Reports indicate that asthma may affect as many as one in every eight children, making it the most common chronic illnesses of childhood. Asthma is a respiratory illness that is characterized by hacking, wheezing, or a shortness of breath. Asthma, if left untreated, may result in asthma attacks, where inflammation and muscle spasms narrow a person's airways.

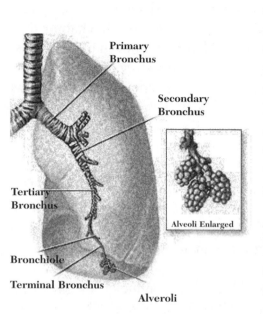

Primary Bronchus

Secondary Bronchus

Tertiary Bronchus

Alveoli Enlarged

Bronchiole

Terminal Bronchus

Alveroli

Nationwide, statistics show there has been a 75 percent increase in asthma cases from 1980 to 1994. Seventeen percent of all emergency department visits are due to asthma. In 1999, 50 percent of children with asthma missed school because of the disease.

"Noni juice has totally controlled my grandson's asthma."

Jan Skelly, a grandmother from Sydney, Australia, proudly relates the effect noni juice had on her grandson's asthma, allergies and ADD.

My grandson, Chad Taylor, has been diagnosed with ADD, has chronic asthma, and is allergic to 80 percent of foodstuffs.

When Chad was 11-years-old he started taking six to seven table-spoons of noni juice every day. Noni juice has totally controlled his asthma. He has rarely needed his steroid puffers since he started taking noni juice in 1998. His food allergies have decreased, and his ADD symptoms are fewer.

We are so grateful to see the changes in Chad. He is happier and so are we! Noni juice has been a great help to him.

In an asthmatic's lungs, the airways called bronchioles constrict abnormally when stimulated by things such as allergens, infections, and exercise. When these bronchioles constrict, it makes it hard to expel air. An x-ray of a person with chronic asthma shows inflammation that is always present. This inflammation results in wheezing, breathlessness, inability to exhale properly, a phlegm or mucus-producing cough, loss of energy, and susceptibility to other respiratory infections.

Health Fact

The number of adults suffering from asthma has more than doubled in the last two decades, with steroid prescriptions increasing six-fold.—*British Medical Journal*

Genetics seems to be one of the major culprits behind asthma as well as an increase in environmental pollutions. Whatever it is that triggers a person's asthma, a food supplement such as noni juice may help in reducing the severity of the symptoms by modulating the immune system and enhancing the cellular structure of the bronchioles. This is, I believe, mostly due to the proxeronine bundled packages sent by the Golgi apparatus and reticuloendothelium to the affected "sick" cells. In addition to asthma caused by allergens, other allergy symptoms such as running nose, itchy eyes, hives, and even eczema have been reduced in many people by drinking noni.

> **"After two days on the noni juice, JC woke breathing and feeling so much better."**
>
> **Nancie Fleming's 15-year-old son, JC, was diagnosed with bronchial asthma. The doctor prescribed steroids, but they used noni juice instead. The results were remarkable.**
>
> *After a severe case of the flu, my son was diagnosed with bronchial asthma. The doctor suggested antibiotics, decongestants, and steroid therapy for seven days. I chose not to give my son any medication. We used only noni juice as his therapy.*
>
> *We used the noni juice therapy every time his allergies to dust, dirt and mold made him sick. The noni juice always gave us excellent results. I started giving JC one ounce of the noni juice every hour for the first eight hours, so eight ounces the first day. The following day he had an ounce every two hours, for a total of six ounces. The next day when JC woke he was breathing and feeling so much better. We continued to give him one ounce of noni juice three times a day for the next few days. His recovery was remarkable!*
>
> *During the summer JC has no allergy symptoms, but when he goes back to school his nose runs and his eyes get red and watery. This year he is drinking one ounce of noni juice as soon as he gets up in the morning, and has not had any of the symptoms of previous years. If he feels a cold coming on we just increase his noni juice until the symptoms are gone. He is a typical teenager, and the extra noni helps him get through any challenges with his health.*

Success Stories
of Noni and Chronic Illness

"My digestive system is perfect, and I am pain free!"

Ken Scanlon, a heavy equipment operator, from Nelson B.C., was only months away from spending the rest of his life in a wheelchair. When he started using noni juice, instead of a wheel chair, he got his health back!

For about 10 years I suffered from a condition of the digestive system that causes bloating and pain in the abdomen. I felt like a guinea pig using all the drugs my doctor prescribed. The drugs damaged my digestive system and made my condition worse. It got so bad my doctor said I would be in a wheelchair within six months.

When a friend introduced me to noni juice, I started using it right away. My symptoms were gone within a month, and I was even able to go back to work! It's been almost two and a half years since I started using noni juice, and I am pain free. My digestive system is perfect, with no more abdominal pain or bloating.

I had another experience with noni juice when I used it topically. Last year a cat scratched my hand. It was a pretty bad scratch, but it was late in the evening and I didn't want to spend hours in the emergency room. I cleaned the wound, but after about half an hour my hand started to swell. My hand got almost the size of a football. It was very painful. That night I soaked my hand in noni juice for about an hour, and I soaked it again in the morning. The infection was gone within twelve hours. I love what noni juice does for me, inside and out!

"I don't know anyone with a candida problem this regimen didn't work for."

April Linkroum suffered with irritable bowel syndrome for almost ten years before finding a regimen that worked. Of course, this therapy included noni juice.

I suffered for almost 10 years with irritable bowel syndrome. Knowing noni juice is anti-fungal, and actually helps good bacteria to grow, I used noni juice with acidophilus and bifidus. The combination was so effective! I no longer have irritable bowel problems, and I don't have to avoid any type of food.

I don't know anyone with a candida problem this regimen didn't work for. I wish I could tell everyone with these kinds of problems about this program. It's amazing how life changing it can be!

"People who haven't seen me recently can't believe I'm the same person."

Doyle Zweifel, a 37-year-old man from Buchman Butte, Saskatchewan, Canada, suffered with kidney problems for years. Before he started taking noni juice the doctors had given him six months to live. Now he is a new man.

I have suffered kidney problems since I was 19, and I've had two kidney transplants. The last transplant was not a perfect match, and I struggled with my body rejecting the kidney. I was on several medications, plus dialysis five times a week. My count was well over 1,000. My blood pressure was 180 over 120. Because of my medical challenges I had been unable to work for a number of years. I was in bad shape and the doctors gave me up to six months to live. When a friend of mine told me about noni juice I decided I didn't have much to lose.

I started drinking six ounces of noni juice a day. I immediately noticed a difference in how good I felt. That was over two and a half years ago and my life has completely changed. I am off all medications, taking dialysis three times a week. Now my count is at 90, and my blood pressure is normal. Because of noni juice my body is even strong enough for another kidney transplant.

Noni has given quality to my life. To me, that means being able to live like a normal person. For the first time in many years I am working 14-16 hours a day. Even after putting in a long workweek, I have the energy to enjoy life. I recently took up golf, and I was able to play four rounds of golf in a tournament.

People who haven't seen me recently can't believe I'm the same person. The transformation has been amazing! I attribute being alive to noni juice. I tell people who are just starting to use noni to give it at least a three-month trial. Otherwise, they won't realize the full effects and they'll be cheating themselves of noni's great benefits.

DIET/NUTRITION RECOMMENDATIONS

When one is suffering from chronic disease, a healthy diet may strengthen the immune system and increase energy levels. Both of these are critical to eventual recovery.

A good diet consists of fruits and vegetables. Eat 15–30 ounces (one to two pounds, or five servings) of a variety of fruits and vegetables daily all year long. Try and eat more vegetables than fruit (about a 65–35 percent ratio), with leafy, green vegetables comprising the significant portion of your vegetable intake.

Other plant foods. Eat approximately seven daily servings of a variety of the following "energy" foods: 1) cereals (but avoiding those that are highly processed), 2) legumes and peas, and 3) roots and tubers.

Alcohol and Tobacco. These are addictive drugs that interfere with the metabolism of many nutrients. They promote poor dietary habits.

Meat (domesticated poultry, fish, beef, pork, and lamb). Try to eat more fish and less red meat.

Fats and oils. Limit consumption of fatty foods, particularly those of animal origin. Choose modest amounts of vegetable oils. These should be mostly polyunsaturated oils, like sunflower or soy oils, or monounsaturated oils, such as olive oil.

Salt. Try to limit consumption of salted foods and the use of extra table salt. Using herbs and spices can do wonders for adding flavor.

SUPPLEMENTATION

There is no way to discuss all of the supplements possible to help with all of the chronic diseases out there. I am including some general supplements that boost overall health.

Vitamin C with bioflavonoids. Vitamin C has been shown time and time again to be a powerful antioxidant (especially when coupled with bioflavonoids).

Essential fatty acids. There are necessary for proper digestion and to maintain energy levels..

Vitamins A and E. Both of these essential vitamins have been shown time and again to aid the body's immune systems.

B-complex vitamins. There is ample research indicating that many B vitamins have a prominent role in helping the body perform the necessary functions to rid itself of disease.

Garlic. Has been shown to help with immune system function.

Chapter Summary Points

- Chronic illness typically "has a long course of illness." However, many people with chronic illness respond positively to extended treatment, both conventional and alternative.

- Noni can positively affect the basic functions of the body, including the metabolism and utilization of each cell in the body, thereby possibly bringing about more energy, particularly in those suffering from CFIDS.

- Noni has been proven to slow down the body's production of the COX 2 enzyme which is a major player in pain and inflammation. Those with fibromyalgia may experience pain relief through a reduction in COX 2.

- A food supplement such as noni juice may help in reducing the severity of the symptoms of asthma by modulating the immune system and enhancing the cellular structure of the bronchioles.

Chapter

8

Diabetes

There is so much more to diabetes than not eating sugar. Diabetes is an all-over body illness. Diabetes is about blindness, skin lesions, kidney failure, nerve damage, headaches, heart failure, fatigue, and yes, even death. Diabetes is the nation's third leading fatal disease, behind only heart disease and cancer. Each year, it is responsible for killing an estimated 150,000 people in the United States alone. The financial costs of diabetes are staggering, resulting in more than $92 billion per year in health-care costs and lost productivity. The emotional costs to those with diabetes as well as to their families and friends can't be measured.

But there is good news. Recent research indicates that diabetes can be controlled and its effects limited. Though there is still no "cure" for diabetes, there is every reason to have confidence and hope that a diabetic can lead a long, active, and productive life. A 10-year national study, completed in 1993, indicated that people with insulin-dependent diabetes, or Type I diabetes, were able to reduce their risk of developing serious long-term complications by 50 percent or more by keeping their blood sugar as close to normal as possible. To a large degree, this can be done simply by modifying the diet to reflect more wise and healthy choices.

Science has revealed how to reduce the risk of serious complications through dietary means. By eating whole, nutritious, natural foods, you may reduce your risk and improve overall health. One food in particular has been shown in historical literature as well as in current studies to possibly further reduce the risks of diabetes and contribute to overall improved health. You guessed it—noni.

"Some Type II diabetics were able to discontinue medications altogether."

Dr. Orlando Pile tells of his own experience and the success he has had with diabetic patients.

In 1997, I finally decided to become a vegetarian. About the same time I heard on the radio about noni, 'the miracle juice.' Initially, I didn't believe what I heard and decided not to follow up. However, for the next two or three months, I continued to hear about noni over the radio. I finally decided to give it a try.

On January 1, 1998, I took my first swallow of noni juice. Needless to say, I didn't like the taste. Nevertheless, I was committed to find out how this juice was going to help me—hopefully by lowering my blood pressure and eliminating my anti-hypertensive medications, or by giving me a so-called burst of energy.

Two months had gone by and I hadn't felt anything. Then, one day while driving with my wife, I was listening to a tape on noni testimonials. "How can this be?" I thought, "Everyone is feeling so wonderful after taking noni, including people's pets, and I'm not feeling anything." At that same moment, my wife asked me about my back condition (referring to my herniated lumbar disk suffered after an auto accident in 1995 and subsequently minimizing my golf playing time). I was so fixed on waiting for a miracle that I never realized my back had stopped hurting. I was so excited that I accepted an invitation to play in a golf tournament in Las Vegas. I took noni before and after playing golf and never had to take one pain killer. For the first time in three years, I was able to play golf without taking a pain pill. At this point I decided to share my experience with my patients in order to hopefully improve their medical conditions.

During this time, I saw Type I and Type II insulin-dependent diabetics lower their insulin doses. Some Type II diabetics were able to discontinue medications altogether.

What is Diabetes?

Diabetes is a disorder of the body that involves the way a body turns food into energy. The problem centers around a substance called insulin, which your body uses to convert food to energy. If your body has diabetes, then your food conversion is all messed up. The body needs food to nourish itself and sustain life. Some foods are better than others. Just like those with severe allergies must avoid those allergens that cause a reaction, so too must diabetics avoid the foods that cause problems.

Food provides both fuel and building material for the body. It produces energy, builds and repairs body tissue, and regulates the manifold body functions and processes. But before food is used by the cells, it has to undergo some biological "steps." First, your body must break down the food you eat into its basic ingredients. These nutrients fall into three major categories—carbohydrates, proteins, and fats.

Carbohydrates, the most abundant of nutrients, are found in most food. Often "starches" and "sugars" are almost completely carbohydrates. Proteins are most abundantly found in meats, poultry, milk, and fish. Fats are found in such foods as vegetable oils, cheese, and other dairy products. All of these nutrients are digested, or broken down, in the stomach and intestines. Carbohydrates are broken down into a simple sugar called "glucose," which is absorbed through the wall of the intestines into your bloodstream. This is what is often called "blood glucose" or, more commonly, just "blood sugar."

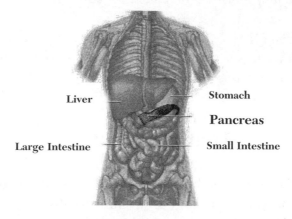

Insulin's Role

Once glucose is absorbed into the bloodstream, it is transported to the body's cells to provide them with the basic unit of energy. But glucose can't simply flow into the cells by itself. Because all cells are enclosed within a thin membrane, something has to tell your cells that glucose is waiting outside. That something is insulin. It attaches on specified sites on the outside of the membrane called insulin receptors—much like a key that fits into a lock. Insulin is the "key" that unlocks the cells, allowing glucose to enter. Once inside, the glucose is metabolized, or "burned," by the cells for energy.

So exactly what is insulin? It is a hormone—a chemical messenger made in one part of the body to transmit "information" via the bloodstream to cells in other parts of the body. Because of the literally thousands of various processes your body needs to operate, the body must then produce many types of hormones. Insulin, made in an organ called the pancreas, is one of these hormones.

During normal digestion, enzymes in the mouth, stomach, and intestines act upon the consumed foods, breaking them down again and again (from carbohydrates, proteins and fats), finally forming them into simple substances, which enter the bloodstream in the following forms:

- Carbohydrates are converted into glucose, which is metabolized or "burned" for quick energy.
- Proteins are converted into amino acids, which provide the basic building blocks for bone, muscle, and other tissue. Proteins also can be burned for energy.
- Fats become fatty acids, which are burned for energy or stored as body fat for potential later use.

Insulin plays a vital role in the burning and storage of all these nutrients. In diabetes, however, its principal role is related to the action of glucose, the simplified form of carbohydrates. Though somewhat simple at first glance, this process is actually complex and amazing. The key players are the beta cells, whose primary responsibility is to make and store the insulin. When the beta cells sense the level of glucose rising in the blood, they respond by releasing just the right amount of insulin into the bloodstream.

As the beta cells first sense a rise in the blood sugar, they release the insulin held in storage. But many times, the body may need even more— this often happens right after a large meal, and as the blood glucose levels increase, a second stage of insulin production begins. The "control centers" of the beta cells trigger them to make even more insulin. As we have mentioned earlier, when functioning normally, the beta cells release just enough insulin to maintain blood glucose levels within the normal range of 60-140 mg/dl. And once in the bloodstream, the insulin allows the glucose to enter your body's cells to use for energy.

There's a bit more to understanding how glucose functions in the body. When you eat, you generally won't need to use all the glucose from your food immediately. So, the body takes some of the glucose and stores it for future need. Later, with the help of insulin, this extra glucose is taken up by the liver cells and changed to a form called "glycogen." Glycogen comes in handy when your body immediately needs extra energy: like during exercise, for example. At these times, your body tries to compensate by quickly changing the stored glycogen back into glucose. In addition, glycogen takes care of your overnight energy needs, a time when you normally aren't eating. Insulin also helps convert some of the extra glucose into fat, which is stored in the body's fat cells.

Diabetes
Fact

About 16 million Americans have diabetes, but only about 10 million have been diagnosed. Approximately 798,000 new cases of diabetes are diagnosed annually in the United States
    —*Centers for Disease Control and Prevention*

What Causes Diabetes?

Diabetes is caused by a breakdown in the normal processes. This can occur in one of two ways: (1) the body produces little or no insulin; or (2) though enough insulin is produced in the body, it can't link with the body's cells. Type I diabetes, or insulin-dependent diabetes, is the result of the first defect; Type II diabetes, called insulin resistant diabetes, is the result of the second. It is important to note, however, that there are some similarities between Type I and Type II diabetes, and that some people display characteristics of both types.

Type I

Of all people with diabetes, only five to ten percent have Type I, which develops most often in children and young adults. That's why it was once called "juvenile-onset" diabetes. However, this type of diabetes can occur in people of any age: thus, we use the term "insulin-dependent" diabetes to describe it. Type I diabetes occurs when the pancreas produces very little, or no insulin. In short, the beta cells cease to function. Individuals who develop Type I diabetes are insulin-dependent. What this means is that they generally must have a daily dose of insulin from an outside source to be able to make use of the food they consume. If they don't, they will cease to function and survive. Usually, insulin is taken by injection with a syringe or with a pump.

Type I diabetes results from the destruction or damage of the beta cells in the pancreas. Why does the body do this? Research has brought us closer to an answer. As yet, scientists don't know for certain. However, as always they have their theories. They believe most diabetic Type I cases are the result of a malfunction in the body's endocrine and immune system.

Symptoms of both Type I and Type II Diabetes

Lack of energy—The body has little or no insulin to enable cells to change blood sugar into energy.

Constant hunger—Unable to get energy from the sugar in your blood, so the body sends out hunger signals for more food.

Weight loss—Unable to use sugar in the blood as a source of energy, the body turns to its fat reserves for energy.

Frequent urination and excessive thirst—Caused by hyperglycemia, or high blood sugar.

Type II

Type II diabetes is the most common kind of diabetes, accounting for approximately 90 percent of all cases. Until recently, Type II diabetes was generally referred to as "maturity-onset" diabetes because it occurs most often in adults 40 years of age or older.

With Type II diabetes, the beta cells still produce insulin, though generally at a reduced rate. A Johns Hopkins Medical research team also found pancreatic antibodies in these patients. In most of such cases, there simply is not enough biologically active insulin to meet the present needs of the body. Type II diabetics usually do not depend on insulin injections to keep basic functions going (though this doesn't mean that they'll necessarily have good health). A number of symptoms are associated with Type II diabetes, many of which are similar to those found with Type I diabetes. However, symptoms may be more subtle in their appearance, thereby making it more difficult for the average person to determine that he/she has Type II diabetes.

Most Type II diabetics are considered insulin resistant. This occurs when the body "resists" taking sugar into its cells. This may happen because: (1) the insulin can't link with the receptors on the surfaces of cells because there aren't enough receptors; or (2) something goes wrong in the chemical reaction at the time of linking. In either situation, the body can't use the sugar in the blood, and high blood sugar develops, bringing on the symptoms of diabetes.

"I will never be out of noni juice."

Barbara Adelaide suffers with asthma, arthritis, and Type II diabetes. After she had been on noni juice for only two months, symptoms from all three ailments were reduced.

I am asthmatic and a Type II diabetic. Since starting on noni juice two months ago, I haven't needed to use my asthma puffer or my nebulizer. My diabetic count has gone down, and I've gone from seven to four prescription pills a day. I have more energy, and I'm not taking as many painkillers for my arthritis. In fact, some days I don't take any pain medication at all!

I am so pleased with the results I've had from noni juice that I've given it to my husband, my three married sons, my mother, and my brother. I will never be out of noni juice! I only wish I had started using it sooner.

Noni and Diabetes

Of the health conditions reported to be helped by noni, diabetes is one of the most common. The historical reports of the island cultures that widely used noni for its medicinal and health promoting properties usually do not refer to diabetes by name. This is probably because these cultures did not know that such a condition existed. However, there are numerous reports of noni helping with symptoms and conditions that accompany both types of diabetes. For instance, noni was commonly reported by the kahunas for treating vision problems, the healing of lingering infections and wounds (signs of a depressed immune system), and to increase energy levels. These are all common symptoms of a diabetic condition.

In our society, there are hundreds of testimonials from doctors, health professionals, and patients that attest to noni's ability to fight diabetes and regulate high blood sugar. Historical use also indicates that noni has long been used as a folk remedy for treating the various symptoms of both types of diabetes, from depressed immune function to fatigue to vision problems.

There are some entirely plausible scientific theories behind noni's mode of action in relieving diabetes, especially of the Type II variety. Since it appears from research at Johns Hopkins Hospital that in diabetes beta cells start to fail in their performance from some sort of autoimmune disorder, this is an area in which we can investigate noni's role in helping with the disease.

A well-tuned immune system typically uses many different cells to carry out the numerous immune functions. These cells are in charge of identifying, killing, and effectively cleaning invading pathogens from the body. However, in the case of autoimmune disorders, the immune system's defense cells turn against the body, attacking perfectly healthy and normally functioning cells. Our research has shown that this is commonly the case with the pancreas' beta cells.

This is where I believe noni comes in. Current studies have revealed that noni has a potent strengthening effect on the immune system, both in enhancing the effect of already functioning immune processes and in stimulating a sluggish immune system. There are a variety of autoimmune disorders that are not well understood or are a total mystery to the medical world. For instance, lupus, fibromyalgia, and chronic fatigue syndrome are all "diseases" whose causes and effects defy precise understanding by doctors and other medical professionals. Yet it is known that these and other conditions are accompanied by a dysfunctioning immune system, resulting in inflammation, pain, and overall discomfort of the joints and other areas of the body. It is quite possible that the beta cells of the pancreas also suffer from the attacking defense cells of the body's immune system in the midst of one of these conditions. Going back to Dr. Anne Hirazumi Kim's research, she has found that noni may modulate the production, activity, and effectiveness of some immune-system agents. These agents are interleukins, interferon, tumor necrosis factor, lipopolysaccharide, and natural killer cells.

"Our patients have also found terrific success using noni"

Psychiatrists Susan Mike, M.D. and her husband, John M. Mike, M.D., tell of their experiences with noni.

We get exposed to all kinds of nutraceuticals on a daily basis. When we heard about noni juice we were skeptical and yet intrigued by the stories we heard from other physicians, nurses, researchers, and natives of French Polynesia. So we investigated the juice ourselves and shared it with our family and friends first.

We were already very healthy. We exercised, ate organic foods, didn't drink or smoke, and we limited our meat intake mainly to fish. The first thing I noticed was that my menstrual cramps were completely gone after two months on the juice. I used to take 800 mg of ibuprofen (that's four tablets) every eight hours for the first two days of my period. After one month on noni, I only used 400 mg and after two months I did not need any ibuprofen. What a relief! My irritability also diminished.

Our families have also had remarkable results with noni. My mother was relieved of her pain from carpal tunnel syndrome in her wrist after only three weeks on the juice (taking only one ounce a day). She has six grandchildren, and three that are under three years old, so she needs full use of her wrists to pick them up and hold them. My uncle experienced relief from chronic gastritis (acid stomach, heartburn). He was in the hospital for a bleeding ulcer two years ago, and now he's pain free and eating peppers, spaghetti sauce, or whatever he wants.

Our patients have also found terrific success using noni for their various conditions. We have seen low and high blood pressure normalize, high cholesterol lower 20 points, diabetes improve to where no pills or less insulin was needed, sleep improve, smoking stop, anxiety diminish, depression lift, and energy and motivation increase.

This is exactly what happened to Joyce's husband, who finally began taking noni after a friend of theirs explained how noni could help him with his diabetes. Joyce explains that "despite his best efforts to take his diabetic medication and keep to a good diet, he could not get his blood sugar levels down below 165 mg/dl (normal is 60-140 mg/dl). However, after taking noni juice for a few short weeks, his glucose levels dropped to a very healthy 100.

Noni consumption may help alleviate diabetic symptoms in other ways. For instance, noni has been shown to stimulate the body's production of two substances—scopoletin and nitric oxide—both known to improve the body's cardiovascular function, thereby reducing conditions that often accompany diabetes. Such conditions include vision problems, poor circulation, retinopathy, and different types of heart disease. Noni also has substantial amounts of fiber, which has a wonderful effect on high blood sugar levels and improves the body's overall digestion and energy utilization processes.

"I did not need as much insulin!"

Gilbert R., a Type II diabetic and bilateral amputee, reduced insulin by 30 percent.

Because I am a diabetic and amputee, I have various health challenges. Not long ago, I was approached by two friends and business associates telling me of something they were involved in—noni juice. To say the least, I was skeptical that it would work, and I was broke. But they convinced me to try it for one month, and after that time if I was not 100 percent satisfied, I could have a full refund.

So, I began taking it immediately. Not more than a few days later, I noticed that I did not need as much insulin! After carefully monitoring my blood sugar, I have been able to safely reduce the amount of insulin I take daily by up to 30 percent. My blood pressure is also the best it has been in years, and I have much more energy than I have had in some time.

Another significant thing that has occurred is that my legs, which both have been amputated, do not hurt as much as they usually do. I have had an open ulcer on the bottom of my left stump for over five years that simply would not heal. Before starting noni, it had opened up to about the size of a silver dollar and was deep enough to go past the second knuckle of my index finger. I have tried numerous things to try and get it to heal. The doctor's last-ditch solution was to take an additional 12 inches off my leg—no, thank you! Since taking the noni, the ulcer has started to close and is now barely the size of a nickel. And I can barely put the end of my finger in!

Complementary Therapies to Noni

DIET/NUTRITION RECOMMENDATIONS

Eat a high-complex-carbohydrate, low-saturated fat, high-fiber diet. This should include plenty of raw vegetables, fruits, and vegetable juices. This will reduce the immediate need for insulin as well as lower the level of fats in the blood. Fiber will also help temper swift surges of blood glucose. Other foods thought to help maintain healthy blood-sugar levels include berries, cheese, egg yolks, fish, garlic, soybeans and soy products, and kelp (often considered a supplement).

Eat frequent, smaller meals throughout the day. This can help reduce the immediate need for a lot of insulin and maintain a lower, more normal blood-glucose level.

Avoid simple carbohydrates. This applies especially to foods high in refined flour and sugar. These result in strong, rapid surges in blood sugar, which usually can't be handled by a diabetic's malfunctioning beta cells. However, when suffering an insulin "reaction," simple sugars can quickly counter the reaction's effects.

Acquire protein from sources such as grains, legumes and other vegetables. Fish and low-fat dairy products are also acceptable sources of protein.

SUPPLEMENTATION

Chromium picolinate. There are numerous studies showing that chromium picolinate can improve the efficiency of insulin utilization, lower blood-sugar levels, reduce the need for diabetes medications, reduce obesity, and enhance the body's ability to use fat for energy.

L-carnitine, L-glutamine and taurine. These amino acids help the body reduce sugar cravings, improve its ability to produce insulin and enhance fat utilization.

Zinc, vanadium, manganese, and magnesium. All of these minerals are known to be involved in the body's maintenance of proper blood-sugar levels.

Vitamin B12. This has been shown to help prevent and even reverse some diabetic neuropathy (damage to nerves that results in sensations of numbness, tingling and pain).

Gymnema sylvestre. This Ayurvedic herb is reported to significantly lower blood-sugar levels.

Quercetin and naringin. These flavonoids can inhibit the activity of the enzyme aldose reductase, which is involved in the development of diabetic cataracts, retinopathy, and neuropathy.

Digestive enzymes. Because the pancreas also produces other substances that contribute to the proper digestion of food, taking digestive enzyme supplements can relieve stress on the body's digestive system.

Bilberry, ginkgo, pycnogenol and hawthorn. These all reportedly help protect the arteries, preventing arteriosclerosis, and slow the development of vascular problems common to diabetics, particularly in the eyes and extremities (hands, toes, fingers, etc.)

Lipoic acid. This helps prevent neuroglycosylation, the adherence of glucose to nerve endings, resulting in pain, numbness, and tingling in various areas of the body.

Essential fatty acids. Because the body is inhibited in its ability to metabolize EFAs, fatty acids such as gamma linolenic acid (GLA) and eicosapentaenoic acid (EPA) are good supplementation investments.

Fiber supplements. Even though improvements in diet can provide the added benefits of more dietary fiber, it is often helpful to add a fiber supplement to one's diet. Fiber helps maintain a more even blood-sugar level for extended periods during the day. Noni is an excellent source of fiber.

OTHER CONSIDERATIONS

Avoid stress. Stress management can play a pivotal role in the treatment of diabetes since uncontrolled and poorly managed tension and anxiety contribute to higher than normal levels of hormones, which negatively affect the actions of insulin. High stress levels can therefore contribute to elevations in blood sugar levels.

Weight management. It is no secret that reducing obesity can help relieve the various symptoms of diabetes, especially fatigue, high blood pressure and poor circulation. Of course, maintaining a proper weight helps counter the development of arteriosclerosis and other forms of heart disease, as well as a host of other debilitating diseases.

Exercise. This goes hand-in-hand with weight management. Exercise can help fight the various forms of heart disease, decrease high blood pressure, lower blood-sugar levels and cholesterol levels, and improve circulation.

Chapter Summary Points

- Diabetes, though a serious condition, can largely be controlled through a healthly diet, careful attention to one's eating habits, a regular exercise program, and other beneficial practices.

- Despite the increase in knowledge of how to diagnose and treat diabetes, more people than ever suffer from the disease.

- Noni has been used historically and in modern times to treat symptoms of diabetes.

- Noni brings help to diabetics through its cellular rebuilding and through increasing the body's consumption of scopoletin. In addition, diabetes is often linked to autoimmune dysfunction (which results in insulin-producing cells becoming damaged or destroyed). By helping modulate the immune system to be more effective, noni helps fight diabetes.

9

Heart Disease

ACE inhibitors, diuretics, lipid-lowering agents—all of these are types of heart medications that have become common, household words. In fact, whether you realize it or not, if you watch an average amount of television chances are you see a commercial for one of these types of medications every day. Why do so many Americans take prescription heart medication like they should be taking our daily vitamin? It's because many are dying from heart disease. In fact, this year alone the Centers for Disease Control and Prevention predict that 700,000 Americans will have a heart attack, despite all our attempts to control the disease through medication.

Heart Disease Fact

About 42 percent of the people who experience a coronary attack in a given year will die from it.
—Centers for Disease Control and Prevention

An incredible 60 million Americans have high blood pressure. The illness, commonly known as hypertension, is the most common reason people go to doctors. It's also the number one health condition for which medication is prescribed in the world today. Add to this figure those who have high cholesterol and those who are obese, and you quickly realize your chance to contract heart disease is awfully high.

Once a person is diagnosed with high blood pressure, he or she is many times more vulnerable to a host of other illnesses and ultimately premature death. For instance, those with hypertension are (on average) seven times more likely to suffer a stroke, four times more likely to have a heart attack, and five times more likely to die of congestive heart failure than healthy individuals.

Heart disease used to be considered a "Western" disease because of this area of the world's high-fat diet, sedentary lifestyle. Add to that smoking, alcohol, and synthetic foods, and you have a recipe for disaster. However, the "Western" world has only been the trend-setter in what has now become a global problem. In the last two years, the World Health Organization (WHO) has confirmed that obesity, diabetes, and heart disease are spreading to the developing world, even in regions suffering from malnutrition. WHO looked at figures from Africa, the Middle East, Latin America, and the Caribbean and saw the all-too-familiar pattern of heart disease and obesity. Some experts say the problem is spreading into third world countries because so is America's industrially produced food. Even in the most remote jungle village it is often easier and less expensive to find a bag of potato chips than it is to find a banana. Urbanization has also made things worse. Cars take a lot less physical energy than bikes or walking. Technology is another culprit. Children who watch television instead playing outdoors learn unhealthy habits early.

There are some areas in the world, however, where blood pressure levels remain within the healthy range throughout a person's entire life. For example, the people of New Guinea and many African nations—even their senior citizens—exhibit blood pressure levels that resemble those of a healthy American teenager. This difference is not based on racial differences. If you were to take those same Africans and feed them the standard American diet, you would see their blood pressures skyrocket to levels that are typical of hypertensive Americans. That is precisely the case among African Americans, 28 percent of whom suffer from high blood pressure and are consuming the ideal diet for hypertension. The disorder also attacks an estimated 16 to 18 percent of white Americans, as well as many Asians, Hispanics, Native Americans, and other ethnic groups.

Around the world, the pattern of heart disease, as well as at its prevention and potential reversal, becomes clear and certain. In most cases, we bring heart disease upon ourselves. Most experts agree that high blood pressure can be reversed in a majority of cases. This can be accomplished through a diet low in fat, cholesterol, salt, and refined foods, coupled with a lifestyle that includes moderate exercise and the maintenance of normal weight. There is also ample evidence to suggest that supplementing with nutraceutical, or natural, agents—just like noni—can contribute to lowering high blood pressure by enhancing the body's ability to battle the condition.

"After being on noni juice for a few short months I had great results."

Joan Chandler now has her blood pressure under control without any medication thanks to noni juice. Pain from a blood clot is gone as well.

When my sister in-law gave me some noni juice I was skeptical, but not for long. After being on noni for a few short months I had great results. I was having trouble with my blood pressure, so I was on medication to keep it under control. Now my blood pressure is at a normal level without any medication. I believe the noni juice is responsible for the improvement.

I had a blood clot in my left calf that caused me a lot of pain. The doctor told me the blood clot had damaged the calf and I would have to live with the pain. My only option was to take anti-inflammatory drugs. I didn't want to take medication on a daily basis, so I gave noni a shot. Thanks to noni juice my leg no longer has any pain—it is healed! Noni juice is a true gift.

What is Heart Disease?

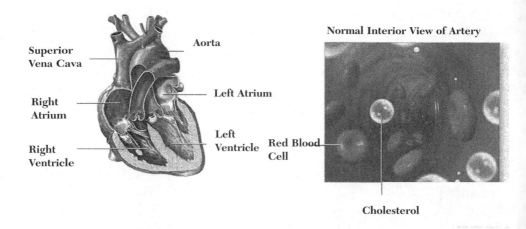

Congestive heart failure, end-stage renal disease, stroke, peripheral arterial disease (clogged vessels in the arms and legs), venous thromboembolism (blood clots), and high blood pressure are all types or symptoms of heart disease.

Stroke and heart attacks are the major causes of death and disability in developed countries, and there are several risk factors that make them more likely to occur. Some are things that we can't do anything about (like age and gender), but the most important are risk factors we can control. The "big three" risk factors are high blood pressure, smoking, and high cholesterol levels. Let's talk about the first and third, since by now we should all know how smoking negatively affects us.

High blood pressure causes damage in several ways. The first is the one most think of initially—the bursting of a blood vessel. Called a stroke, this usually occurs in the brain when a small artery develops a weak spot and eventually breaks. High blood pressure also negatively affects the body in the undue strain it puts on the heart. Because the heart has to work excessively to do its job, it grows, just like any other muscle that is used excessively. People that don't have high blood pressure, such as athletes, may also have an enlarged heart, but theirs is due to the increased amount of blood needed to accommodate their activity. People with high blood pressure, on the other hand, don't need a larger volume of blood, they simply need to push the blood they have through smaller, non-elastic vessels. This leads to thicker heart walls, which is bad because the heart then outgrows its own blood supply.

The third big risk factor, high cholesterol, may cause the deposition of cholesterol plaque in the arteries. This may take years to develop, but it is very difficult to detect until it causes a major blockage. These deposits can occur in the heart, causing heart attacks and angina (severe pain); the kidneys, where it causes renal failure and even higher blood pressure; the brain, where it causes strokes; and the legs, resulting in a condition known as intermittent claudication, which is pain while walking.

"Every year the cycle started over with cluster headaches bothering me from January to May."

Clint Wilkinson a dentist, was 42-years-old when cluster headaches took over his life. Very skeptically he tried noni juice, and within two days his headaches were gone!

I began suffering from cluster headaches five years ago. I had no idea what I was in for when I woke up in the middle of the night on February 1, 1998. I felt like someone was scraping the back of my right eye socket with a spoon. This went on for hours. The pain returned a few hours later, lasting several more hours. These headaches bothered me six to eight times a day for three months.

I was a 42-year-old dentist with a very busy practice. Suddenly I was unable to work any kind of predictable schedule, due to the severity of my headaches. I literally could not think in the middle of them. I thought I would go crazy with the pain.

I went to the Mayo Clinic in Jacksonville, Florida, where my neurologist's diagnosis of "Cluster Headaches" was confirmed. I was told they might last several months, or become chronic, never going away. I was given a blood pressure medication and some painkillers, but nothing worked. Every year the cycle started over. The headaches began at the end of January, and continued through the beginning of May.

This year the clusters came on January 31. I went to my neurologist, and had an IV infusion of steroids on three separate days. This treatment only made things worse, because I was unable to sleep for nearly four days, and I still had the headaches.

At the end of the week, with my life going into a tail spin again, a friend told me about noni juice. He said it worked on migraine headaches and a lot of other conditions as well. I objected to the idea; nothing works on everything. And besides, I reasoned, cluster headaches have a different mechanism than migraines.

"What do you have to lose?" he challenged me.

In desperation I gave noni a try. I started drinking two ounces of noni juice in the morning and two more ounces in the evening. Within two days my headaches were gone, never to return! In addition, I began sleeping better. Within a week my energy level was higher than it has been in 20 years. As I've continued taking noni juice I have become more resistant to upper respiratory tract infections, and I've seen an improvement in my irritable bowel syndrome. My generalized body aches have even disappeared. Maybe noni juice does work on everything!

Blood Pressure Blues

At the core of the cardiovascular system is the heart. From the heart branch off the arteries, which are the principal pipeline for the blood carried from the heart to various tissues and organs. They are configured like a tree: the central trunk, or aorta, leaves the heart and then branches repeatedly. Eventually, the blood vessels branch into arterioles, very small vessels that are visible only under a microscope. Arterioles have muscle cells in their walls, allowing them to constrict and dilate just like the main arteries, and therefore contribute to the control and direction of blood flow to where it is most needed. The arterioles branch into even finer vessels, called capillaries, which form a delicate mesh that supplies the tissues with oxygen and other nutrients. For the blood to be able to circulate properly, a certain level of pressure is needed to force it through the arterioles and capillaries.

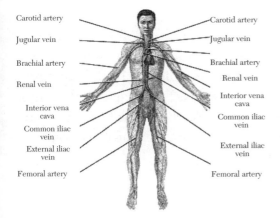

Carotid artery
Jugular vein
Brachial artery
Renal vein
Interior vena cava
Common iliac vein
External iliac vein
Femoral artery

Carotid artery
Jugular vein
Brachial artery
Renal vein
Interior vena cava
Common iliac vein
External iliac vein
Femoral artery

It's important to realize that our blood pressure is continually varying in order to meet the changing needs of our bodies. In fact, some of us have high blood pressure some of the time, and we wouldn't be able to function well if we didn't. However, when high blood pressure is sustained for long periods of time it becomes a health concern. The changes in blood pressure were noted for real the first time that blood pressure was measured. In 1733, an English priest named

Stephen Hales inserted a glass tube into a major neck artery of a horse, and was surprised to see that the blood reached a height of about eight feet in the tube. Not surprisingly, the horse didn't much enjoy having a glass tube stuck into its neck, so its ensuing struggle brought about an increase in its blood pressure, evidenced by a sharp rise of blood in the glass tube.

Blood pressure is the force exerted on the blood as it moves through your arteries. The force of the pumping heart muscle against the resistance of the blood vessels creates the "pressure." Your blood pressure rises and falls naturally throughout the day. When you wake up, get out of bed, exercise, or experience stressful situations, your heart beats more rapidly to meet the increased demand for blood and oxygen from cells and tissues throughout the body. This increase in heart rate also increases your blood pressure during these particular times. Blood pressure falls while you rest, and especially while you sleep, because the demands on the heart are greatly diminished. In healthy people, blood pressure rises when heart rate increases, and drops into the normal ranges when the increased demand is relieved.

What the Numbers Mean

Generally, blood pressure is expressed in numbers as a fraction, such as 120/85. Two numbers are used because there are two pressures being measured. The first pressure, called systolic, is indicated by the top number, and it represents the phase when the heart contracts and pumps blood into the aorta, the body's main artery. As the blood is pushed into the arteries, they expand. The recoil of those arteries, or their contraction, creates the second type of blood pressure, called diastolic. This pressure occurs while the heart rests, the valves open, and the ventricles fill with blood. While the heart expands, the arteries contract and serve as a kind of second pumping action.

Diastolic pressure, therefore, indicates the relative flexibility of your arteries. The less flexible your arteries are the more pressure they will exert as they recoil on the blood. It's a lot easier for the heart to pump blood through soft, flexible arteries than to pump blood through hard, inflexible vessels. The degree of inflexibility of those arteries indicates how much resistance the heart must overcome to pump the blood. Naturally, the harder the vessels, the harder the heart must work.

White-Coat Hypertension

Have you ever gone to the doctor and had to wait an hour with crying children in the waiting room before you were ushered to see the doctor? The stress and tension of going to the doctor is enough to make some people's high blood pressure abnormally rise. Blood pressure readings are usually higher when taken at a doctor's office. This phenomenon is commonly referred to as "white-coat hypertension." Anyone with high blood pressure, even if it is mild, should buy a home high-blood pressure cuff. By checking your pressure regularly at home, you will get more consistent and accurate reading.

A healthy blood pressure reading depends largely on the individual. A common rule of thumb is that a blood pressure below 140/90 is normal, and that a pressure above 160/100 is too high and considered dangerous. The resulting gray area, where there is genuine disagreement among doctors, is the blood pressure area that falls between these two ranges. My personal feeling is that blood pressure should be kept below 125/85, preferably 110/76 or lower.

High blood pressure is usually a symptom of some other underlying condition. People with high blood pressure usually do not appear or feel sick. They function quite well. It's only when blood pressure gets to very high levels (malignant hypertension) that it makes people feel sick. For the majority with only "moderate" hypertension, the danger is in the wear and tear on the cardiovascular system.

How Noni Helps Lower High Blood Pressure

There are a number of ways in which noni may help reduce high blood pressure. First, noni contains a substance called scopoletin, which has been scientifically proven to help constricted blood vessels dilate, thereby lowering blood pressure. Another reason noni may be able to help relieve high blood pressure is because of its stimulatory effect on the body's production of nitric oxide. Nitric oxide (NO) has been shown to have a positive effect on allowing blood vessels to be more elastic, resulting in lower blood pressure and an overall beneficial effect on the entire cardiovascular system.

"I'm jumping with joy. I am so very thankful for the benefits of noni juice!"

Mary Grace was able to clear up a serious uterine condition in less than four months time using only noni juice.

Five months ago I was diagnosed with a uterine condition that causes the walls of the uterus to become inflamed. This is often due to menopause and in many cases the precursor to more serious conditions, including cancer. Medication was prescribed and lab work was scheduled every three weeks. The first lab results showed the condition was still prevalent and I had to increase my medication to three times weekly. That was approximately the same time I began using noni juice. Initially, I drank two ounces in the morning, and then increased to two ounces twice daily.

On my next visit the doctor reported the walls of my uterus were "thickening"—a sign of improvement and healing. I increased my doses of noni and decreased my medication to only once a week. Three weeks later the lab results showed that I still had some slight inflammation; however, there was improvement overall. Once again labs were ordered three weeks later. Today, I am happy to report those results came back showing my Pap smear completely normal.

Another benefit I attribute to noni juice: My doctor has advised me I can reduce the blood pressure medication I've been taking for over 10 years. I'm jumping with joy, and I am so very thankful for the benefits of noni juice!

Scopoletin

Though discovered some time ago, scopoletin was only isolated from noni extract in 1993 by researchers at the University of Hawaii. There is an impressive body of data that reveals scopoletin's antihypertensive properties. Despite this valuable capability, there are some who have expressed concern over indications that scopoletin may occasionally lower blood pressure to below-normal levels. However, in all of the research, the thousands of case studies, and the files of user feedback that I have reviewed, I have yet to come across one documented case in which noni lowered blood pressure to below-normal levels.

One may ask how this is possible, seeing that noni contains scopoletin, and scopoletin has been shown to occasionally cause low blood pressure. I believe it is possible for a number of reasons. First, in most botanicals that demonstrate medicinal benefits, there are a number of biochemicals, compounds, and other substances that work synergistically (enhancing each other's properties while simultaneously preventing side effects) to create the desired health benefit. In the case of noni, I believe this to be true.

This brings us to another explanation of how scopoletin may help lower high blood pressure without taking it too low. Think back to the Golgi apparatus. The role of this mini "post office" is to package together specific amounts of various substances—hormones, biochemicals, vitamins, amino acids, fats, and other nutrients such as scopoletin—and "mail" them to the cells (or parts of cells) that need the package of nutrients in order to maintain or regain normal function.

"My doctor wants all the information I can give him!"

Joan Chandler shared her health improvements with her doctor and his staff. Now, they want to know more!

I have noticed several improvements in my health since I started taking noni juice. I haven't had to take any blood pressure medication since I started drinking the noni, and all my seizures are gone. I haven't had any more asthma attacks, and the pain I was having in my left calf, due to a blood clot, is gone!

Thanks to noni I'm doing great! I told my doctor about noni juice and what it has done for my health. He wants all the information I can give him! All the nurses in his office want to know about noni and weight loss.

Nitric Oxide

Nitric oxide is important in the body's maintenance of a smooth-running cardiovascular system. Dr. Anne Hirazumi Kim, in her studies on cancer, has postulated that noni stimulates the body's production of nitric oxide. While the principal study investigating noni and nitric oxide focused on NO's ability to fight cancerous cells, it is no leap of logic to assume that nitric oxide stimulated by the presence of noni extract could also be used to fight high blood pressure and contribute to an improved and healthy heart and vascular system.

So how does NO lower blood pressure? Many researchers now believe that nitric oxide may be at the core of the somewhat complex process of regulating blood pressure. Essentially, endothelium cells produce and release nitric oxide into the bloodstream, which in turn causes the smooth muscles making up the vessel walls to relax, ultimately leading to a more normal elasticity in the blood vessels, less wear and tear on the heart, and a lower, healthier blood pressure.

The treatment of high blood pressure with nitric oxide makes perfect theoretical sense, given the dual benefits of relaxing arteries and inhibiting blood clots. But does it really work in real patients? Yes! Here are a few samplings from recently collected data:

- The study conducted by Dr. Anne Hirazumi and colleagues from the University of Hawaii clearly shows that noni extract enhances the production of nitric oxide in the endothelial cells. Though the study focused more on nitric oxide's role in fighting cancerous and other invasive organisms, the ramifications are clear. Couple this with the widespread reports that noni has a definite positive effect on high blood pressure, and it is clear that noni (and specifically, noni-induced nitric oxide) encourages the dilation of constricted blood vessels, thereby relieving hypertension and benefiting the cardiovascular system in other ways as well.

- A recent clinical trial consisted of hypertensive men ranging in ages from 35 to 65 who volunteered to withdraw from blood pressure medication for one week. Each morning, they were given intravenous arginine (an amino acid known to stimulate the body's production of nitric oxide). This injection created a rapid decrease in both systolic and diastolic blood pressure in all the patients, an effect that lasted about 20 minutes. No other symptoms other than dry mouth were reported.

- Another study revealed that five patients with hypertension were given intravenous arginine. They had an average high blood pressure of 154/95 mm Hg before treatment, but shortly afterwards, their systolic pressure dropped an average of nearly 30 mm Hg and the diastolic pressure decreased an average of 22 mm Hg.

- Scott Gerson, M.D., of the Mt. Sinai School of Medicine in New York, completed a placebo-controlled clinical trial to determine whether noni really could lower high blood pressure. For 14 weeks, Dr. Gerson studied nine hypertensive patients—six males and three females. These patients were selected at random, and did not know that they were taking a noni extract. They stayed on the same diet and maintained the same exercise regimens previous to their beginning the trial. After 14 weeks of noni treatment, eight of the nine patients showed a significant decrease in blood pressure. On average, their systolic pressure (which is the number read on top) dropped by almost 8 percent, and their diastolic pressure (the bottom number) decreased 4 percent.

I have received exciting reports from various doctors who regularly suggest noni as a natural treatment for high blood pressure. The late Dr. Mona Harrison detailed the account of one of her patients, who had suffered from high blood pressure. Her doctors had been able to lower it to about 170/100, but no more. Turning to Dr. Harrison, she was encouraged to take noni juice. After only two months of taking noni, her blood pressure dropped to a normal, healthier level of 130/80.

Catching up to Cholesterol

Cholesterol is a soft, waxy substance found in the bloodstream and in the body's cells. It's normal to have cholesterol; in fact, it's an important part of a healthy body because it's used for producing cell membranes. The adage, "Too much of a good thing is never a good thing" applies here. Hypercholesterolemia is the technical word for high levels of blood cholesterol.

If you have high cholesterol, there are two things possibly happening inside your body. First, every person's body naturally makes cholesterol. Some who have high cholesterol readings simply may have a system that is out of whack and is making too much cholesterol. A second possibility is that the body is gleaning extra cholesterol from the fats in the animal products that you eat, such as meats, poultry, fish, eggs, butter, cheese and milk. This is typically the way that most people end up with high cholesterol

Cholesterol doesn't dissolve in the blood. Instead, cholesterol has to be hauled around by special carriers called lipoproteins. The two most common kinds are low-density lipoprotein, or LDL, and high-density lipoprotein, or HDL. LDL is known as the carrier for bad cholesterol, or the cholesterol headed toward the arteries. HDL carries around the good cholesterol, or the cholesterol that is headed away from the arteries. Studies suggest that high levels of HDL cholesterol reduce your risk of heart disease, while high levels of LDL increase your risk.

In the chapter on arthritis, we talked in detail about the discovery of the COX 2 enzyme and how it related to noni and inflammation pain. However, arthritis is not the only disease in which the COX 2 enzyme has been implicated. Cancer, Alzheimer's and even high cholesterol all have a connection with the COX 2 enzyme.

Originally discovered by a researcher studying cancer, the COX 2 enzyme oxidizes or burns up a fat in the body called "arachidonic acid." This fat is an omega-6 fatty acid, and it occurs naturally in all of the cell walls. COX 2 works by igniting the fat and burning it up. The inflammation is a by-product of this "burning." The COX 2 enzyme actually has a useful purpose in the body. The body uses COX 2 in response to a bacterial infection or to trauma and injury. However, in many people the body starts to use too much COX 2, or the body may use the enzyme sporadically to burn up the cell's "arachidonic acid" for no reason. The body's uncontrolled use of COX 2 can cause inflammation in all parts of the body ranging from the joints (as seen with arthritis) to the neurons found within the brain (as seen with Alzheimer's), as well as in the blood, as with cholesterol. Let me explain.

In an immune system that is functioning out of control, not only are bacterial and viral infections sought out and destroyed, but so are normal blood particles that are supposed to be present, such as HDL cholesterol, or the good kind of cholesterol. Studies show that cholesterol can trigger a low-level inflammation response from an overactive immune system. This low-level inflammation may go unnoticed for years. However, this inflammation disturbs even small build-ups of plaque, which can eventually make them rupture from the artery walls and cause a blood clot. Researchers believe this may be why people with only average amounts of cholesterol can suddenly have a heart attack. Sometimes, it's not the level of cholesterol that is the problem, but the presence of low-level inflammation. That is why by controlling the COX 2 enzyme the precursor to inflammation you help in preventing heart disease.

The ideal situation is to find a substance that inhibits the COX 2 enzyme while minimizing the inhibition of the COX 1 enzyme, a good enzyme that protects the lining of the stomach. Scientific findings from carefully conducted research done in an independent laboratory confirmed that TAHITIAN NONI ® Juice reduces the amount of COX 2 while allowing the body to continue producing COX 1, thereby possibly helping those with arthritis, some genetic cancers, brain inflammation, and yes, even high cholesterol.

"He hasn't had any discomfort in his chest since the surgery!"

Sharon Boniek, shares her husband's great recovery after open heart surgery. He was taking noni juice before the surgery, while in the hospital, and when he returned home. They feel that the noni juice made the difference.

At 75 years of age, my husband Elmer came through his open-heart surgery with flying colors! The doctors and nurses were quite amazed at how well he did and how jovial he was afterwards.

While he was in the hospital I took him a little bit of noni juice every day. I am amazed he hasn't had any discomfort in his chest area since the surgery! He has never taken any pain medication at home.

He is gaining new strength every day. He takes about a six-ounce bottle of noni to bed. He drinks in the night when he wakes, plus more during the day. We are so grateful for the noni juice. I know it has kept him strong, helps him recuperate, and will give me back my strong and energetic husband!

Complementary Therapies to Noni

As part of a holistic health plan, noni can provide substantial benefits in lowering high blood pressure and improving the health of the heart and cardiovascular system. But there are other regimens that can enhance noni's function in fighting hypertension. The following provide other legitimate therapies and treatments for treating high blood pressure and the pursuit of overall improved health.

DIET/NUTRITION RECOMMENDATIONS

Change your diet. Diet is probably the most important factor in both preventing and treating hypertension. Incorporate a diet that is low in high-fat red meat, dairy products, and processed sugar/flour products, and high in whole foods, coldwater fish, and lean white meats. Consume plenty of oat bran, pectin-containing fruits and vegetables, and other fresh fruits and vegetables, including broccoli, cabbage, green leafy vegetables, peas, prunes, beets, and carrots (there are other great options, of course). The incidence of high blood pressure is considerably lower in vegetarians.

Reduce salt intake to moderate levels. Salt encourages the retention of fluid, which contributes to rising blood pressure.

Avoid caffeine. This can temporarily (yet unnecessarily) raise blood pressure.

Increase consumption of garlic and onions. Garlic has been shown to be effective in lowering blood cholesterol levels, as well as in bringing down blood pressure readings. Because many people believe they don't get enough garlic in their diet, they opt for supplementation. Odorless garlic capsules are recommended. Onions provide some of the same benefits as garlic.

Incorporate celery into your diet. Consuming celery, and specifically celery seed and celery oil, has been linked to lowering blood pressure. Celery seed has been used for generations by folk healers and Chinese physicians in the treatment of high blood pressure.

Use more olive and flaxseed oil. If used for cooking and baking purposes, these oils have a health-promoting effect rather than health-degrading effect. Decrease the use of hydrogenated fats (like margarine).

Eliminate certain foods. Avoid smoked and aged cheeses and meats, chocolate, animal fats, gravies, some canned soups, diet soda, meat tenderizers, soy sauce and ibuprofen medications. These all contain substances, such as monosodium glutamate, that have been linked to high blood pressure and other cardiovascular disease.

SUPPLEMENTATION

Essential fatty acids. Found in fish oils and other plant oils like flaxseed and borage, fatty acids can contribute to the reduction of both high blood pressure and blood lipids. Remember that if you are taking a fish oil supplement, it is also wise to take a vitamin E supplement.

Vitamin C with bioflavonoids. Studies have shown that supplementing with vitamin C and bioflavonoids may reduce blood pressure. These are compounds that act as free radical scavengers in the arteries and heart muscle.

Fiber supplement. It is well known that the average American does not get enough dietary fiber, so a fiber supplement can help make up the deficit. Studies show that boosting fiber intake can be a very effective method in treating both high blood pressure and high blood cholesterol levels.

Calcium/magnesium. There is a large body of research linking the deficiency of these two substances to high blood pressure.

Selenium. Deficiencies of this mineral have also been linked to high blood pressure and heart disease. Because most diets are lacking in this mineral, supplementation may be vital.

Herbal combination containing cayenne, chamomile, fennel, hawthorn berries and rosemary. These and other herbs have been used for centuries to treat the various symptoms of heart disease.

Valerian, hops and kava. These three herbs can help relieve anxiety, which can play a role in high blood pressure.

Coenzyme Q10. This valuable substance has been shown to possess multiple health benefits, among them improving the health of the heart and related tissues. It has also been shown to help lower hypertension.

OTHER RECOMMENDATIONS

Don't smoke. As we discussed earlier in the chapter, smoking is one of the "big three" factors for increasing the risk of stroke and heart attack. It also goes without saying that not smoking produces a number of other health benefits as well.

Get rid of excess weight. Another of the "big three" risk factors for stroke and heart attack, being overweight can be dealt with in various ways, diet and exercise being the most effective. There are numerous studies proving that excess weight dramatically increases one's risk of developing hypertension and other related cardiovascular conditions, and premature death.

Implement a stress-reduction program. An impressive body of research reveals that relieving stress can significantly reduce high blood pressure levels. Meditation techniques can diffuse stress, leading to lower blood pressure. Other therapies, such as relaxation techniques and exercise, can significantly reduce mental and emotional stress, which can ultimately lead to a more normal blood pressure.

Exercise. This one is simple: exercising for at least a half hour, three times weekly, can do wonders for high blood pressure. It has numerous other benefits as well.

Have your blood pressure checked regularly. This can be done either at home or by your doctor, and will help you track your progress in improving your condition.

Chapter Summary Points

- Heart disease is the Western world's number one killer, and it is spreading to underdeveloped parts of the world as well. Factors such as high-fat diets, sedentary lifestyles, and high stress lead to problems with the cardiovascular system.

- Because high blood pressure can be largely controlled through special attention to diet, exercise and other factors, noni may help lower high blood pressure if incorporated into a holistic health plan.

- The big three risk factors are high blood pressure, smoking, and high cholesterol. Noni has been shown to help with high blood pressure and high cholesterol in particular as they relate to heart disease.

- There is research indicating that noni either contains or stimulates the production of a number of substances than can help lower high blood pressure. Most notable among these are scopoletin and nitric oxide, both of which are proven antihypertension agents.

- COX 2 enzyme inhibitors such as noni, have also been shown useful in maintaining a healthy LDL/HDL cholesterol ratio.

Chapter
10
Infections

A hundred years ago, the leading cause of death was from infectious diseases such as polio, measles, and tuberculosis. Nowadays, chronic disease has taken over as the number one killer; however, invaders such as bacteria, viruses, fungi and parasites are still around. These pesky pathogens are responsible for a multitude of our most common health complaints like colds, flu, upset stomach, and the like. They can range in seriousness from the common cold to flesh-eating bacteria.

In older days, things such as an infected sliver or an abscessed tooth could ruin a person's life. Without modern-day antibiotics, things of that nature were not only painful, but life-altering. In response to these threats, medical healers throughout the ages have looked for effective ways to fight infection. Noni has been used for centuries for various health problems, including infections, by numerous cultures worldwide.

"Noni finally took care of this horrible problem."

Paula Moore had toenail fungus for years. She tried everything to get rid of it with little success until noni.

I've had toenail fungus for years! I tried everything. Noni finally took care of this horrible problem. Now I'm putting noni on my fingernails to help strengthen them. Because it's antibacterial it is beneficial in other ways as well.

This historical use of noni for infection is prolific. The Polynesians utilized the whole noni plant in many of their medicinal remedies. Noni's root, stem, bark, leaves, flowers, and fruit are all involved in various combinations in almost 40 known and recorded herbal remedies, many of which remedies were for the treatment of infection. The fruit was so popular that a Tongan myth tells of the god Maui being restored to life by having noni leaves placed on his body. Numerous other historical accounts back noni's ability to fight bacterial and viral invaders. From Guam to India to the West Indies, noni has been used to treat infected ulcers, wounds, boils, skin diseases, sinus infections, and other problems caused by infection.

Modern research supports the historical use of noni as an antimicrobial agent. One of the very first medical articles about noni comes from a man named Allen who reported on the ethnobotanical properties of noni. His work described noni as deobstruent (or something that has the power to clear and open ducts and secretions of the body). Another medical article by Bushnell reports that noni was a traditional remedy used to treat broken bones, deep cuts, bruises, sores, and wounds.

In 1950, researchers in the journal *Pacific Science* reported that noni fruit possessed antibacterial properties against several bacterial strains: P. aeruginosa, M. pyrogenes and E. coli. University of Hawaii researcher Oscar Levand also found noni fruit extract to have remarkable abilities to ward off infection from several bacterial species, including Salmonella typhosa, Pseudomonas aeruginosa, Proteus morganii, Staphylycoccus aureus, Bacillus subtilis and Escherichia coli (E. coli).

More recently, Joseph Betz, a research chemist in the FDA's Division of Natural Products, Center for Food Safety and Applied Nutrition, reports that noni has been tested for a number of biological activities, some of which activities are related to infection.

Botanist Julia Morton reports that noni has been used in the Philippines as a vermifuge (an agent that aids the body in expelling parasites) and for relieving such conditions as boils, carbuncles, and stomach ulcers (often caused by the bacteria *H. pylori*) in Hawaii. She also notes that noni was used to treat ringworm, boils, ulcers, wounds, and as a potent insecticidal wash.

One modern story, which I received from a woman named Maren, told how her eight-year-old niece had been suffering from chronic bladder infections. Things had become so bad that her doctor decided to put her on a low-dose antibiotic for a few months. This troubled the girl's parents, so they decided to start giving her noni. On a Sunday they gave her one tablespoon of noni juice, and followed with a similar dose for the next four days. On Thursday, the doctor took another blood test, which yielded a negative result. Furthermore, the girl's symptoms were almost entirely absent. She has been taking noni consistently ever since, and has had no problems with her bladder infections.

"*I became committed to noni juice.*"

Phil Zamora was diagnosed HIV positive in 1988. He started using noni juice in 2002, and is now off all HIV drugs. He wants to share his experience with noni juice so it may help others with HIV.

I was diagnosed HIV positive in 1988. I was a professional musician, and the touring lifestyle and the 'fast lane' took its toll on my health. November 11th, 1987 I stopped drinking and using all recreational drugs. I started a new life with a good wholesome diet, some good vitamins and herbal supplements, and the support of the 12-step program. Even with all the positive changes I made I couldn't turn back the clock. I developed full-blown AIDS in January of 1997 and was given a slim to no chance of survival at UCSF Medical Center in San Francisco. Due to the fact I was clean and sober with a strong will to live, I pulled through with the help of newly discovered drugs. The side effects, caused by the toxicity of HIV drugs, were unbearable. Since 1998 I've struggled with the virus mutating, and having to change drugs frequently. At one point I was suffering from so many side effects, I told the doctors to just let me die quickly instead of suffering.

In 2000 I met a woman at work who had a bottle of noni juice in the break room. I thought she was bringing a bottle of wine to work, and I was going to "12-step" her about her drinking problem. After a good laugh I found that it was noni juice. She told me what a great health drink it was and gave me a shot. My production level that day increased two fold, and my memory seemed to sharpen. However, it wasn't until later that I became committed to noni juice.

In 2002 I was having problems, once again, with side effects and another mutation of HIV. The doctor told me there were no drugs left to combat the HIV, and I'd better stick to the drug program or I would die. I decided to give noni a try in a serious way. I started drinking four to eight ounces of noni juice a day for three weeks. Then I decreased my dose to three to four ounces a day for a few weeks. My blood work came back from 145 t-cells to where it is now, almost 400 with a non-detectable viral load.

My wife contracted HIV from me, and after watching me wean away from my HIV medications she decided to try the noni juice. She started with three shots a day. Her last major blood work in February of 2003 went from 600 to almost 1,000!

I am now completely off the "meds from hell," using noni juice as my only medication. I will be introducing this great healing juice to the staff at the Positive Health Department of UCSF in San Francisco. I hope to give the doctors a helping hand in the healing of AIDS. I would like them to consider noni juice as an alternative to HIV medications that take away dignity and good living while draining our pockets.

Tuberculosis

While tuberculosis is no longer a major health threat in most areas in the United States, it is still a problem in less developed areas of the world. The cases of tuberculosis that do resurface seem to be from drug-resistant strains that don't respond to usual anti-microbial treatment. For these two reasons, researchers have been looking for new ways to combat the disease.

At the 2000 International Chemical Congress of Pacific Basin Societies hosted by American Chemical Society, researchers from the University of Santo Tomas in Manila, Philippine Islands, presented a study that showed noni had been found to kill the bacterium *tuber bacillus,* which causes tuberculosis.

In the Philippine study, Dr. Jonel Saludes and others found that in laboratory tests a concentration of extracts from the leaves of the noni plant killed 89 percent of the pathogens known to cause tuberculosis. The leading tuberculosis drug currently used, rifampicin, killed 97 percent of the pathogens at comparable concentrations. That means noni was only 8 percent less effective than a synthetic drug with possible negative side effects.

The active compounds in noni that researchers believe are responsible for the inhibition activity of tuberculosis pathogens are the phytosterols within noni (otherwise known as plant sterols). Noni's phytosterols are structurally different from the other compounds used to treat tuberculosis. Because of this, researchers believe that the compounds within the noni extract are fighting off the pathogens using a different mechanism than the traditional drugs use. (Plant sterols are safe and shouldn't be confused with "steroids" used in humans.)

These researchers, funded by the Philippine government, the International Foundation for Science, and UNESCO, say that the results are very promising. As a result, they will continue to study the plant, and they encourage pharmaceutical companies to do the same. The team indicated that studies of the different parts of the plant, such as the fruit, are under way.

"Leland is even growing new hair on the top of his head!"

Leland and Alice Strommen tried noni juice together. Alice shares their life-changing results:

My sinus problems stopped within just a few days of starting noni juice, and my lungs are much clearer. The cloudy film over my eyes is gone—a symptom that has bothered me for years. It is wonderful to see clearly again!

In the past, whenever I traveled I would get sick as soon as I arrived at my destination, and I remained so until several days after I'd returned home. I have taken several trips since starting on the noni juice and I haven't gotten sick once!

I suffer from arthritis and have been on pain medications for many years. I am now free of all pain and pain medication.

My husband and I are more mentally alert, and we feel better. Both of our gray hair has gotten darker, and Leland is even growing new hair on the top of his head! (That is exciting for any man.) We no longer crave sweets—I've even lost a few inches!

Noni juice is such a wonderful product and has been a blessing to our lives.

Infection's No. 1 Enemy—The Immune System

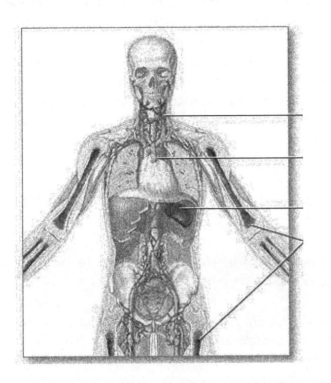

Lymph Nodes

Thymus

Spleen

Long Bones

In addition to these compounds within noni that fight against infection, Dr. Anne Hirazumi Kim's research shows how noni may work to fight infection by modulating the unique system in the body that naturally fights disease. Her study from the University of Hawaii reports noni modulates the production of various immune agents, including nitric oxide, interleukin 1, interleukin 2, interleukin 4, interleukin 10, interleukin 12, interferon, and lipopolysaccharide, most of which help fight many pathogens, whether they be viral, bacterial, cancerous, parasitic, or fungal. Another recent study also indicates that scopoletin, a health-promoting agent found in noni, may inhibit the activity of E. coli, commonly associated with recent outbreaks resulting in hundreds of serious infections and even death.

These and other studies provide exciting data indicating that noni can indeed aid the body in stimulating and strengthening its various immune functions, thereby adding valuable protection against pathogenic agents like bacteria, viruses, cancerous cells, fungi and parasites. Noni's principal method of helping defend against these infectious agents is its immunostimulatory ability. In other words, noni possesses the ability to stimulate or encourage the production, even above normal levels, of the already listed immune fighting cells. In turn, these cells are the primary force behind ridding the body of unwanted invaders.

"I felt like someone had literally lifted the curtain and I walked out of the fog."

Nancie Fleming tells her amazing story using noni to relieve her battle with shingles.

I suffered for over two and a half years with shingles. The shingles bothered me for about nine months in my left arm. One day I was relieved when they disappeared, only to have them reappear in my right arm. They bothered me there for another nine months. Then they returned to my left arm for ten more months. During that time I tried many treatments—both medical and alternative—with no relief.

In October 1996 my friend introduced me to noni juice. I started to drink one ounce of noni juice three times a day. Within three days my energy level increased 10 times. By the seventh day I was finally sleeping through the night—something I hadn't done for two and a half years. I felt like someone had literally lifted a curtain and I walked out of the fog. It was incredible! On the 14th day of taking noni juice I broke out in a rash all over the top of my chest and down my arms. I knew the noni juice must have been working. Twenty-four hours later my rash was gone—and so were my shingles!

It is now September 2000, almost four years later, and I have noticed many other health conditions disappear. A 15-year chronic lower-back problem is better. After drinking noni juice for about a year I noticed the blue spider veins I've had for 25-year-old up the back of both legs were gone. The headaches I suffered with almost daily have vanished. If I feel like I'm getting the flu or a headache I simply take some extra noni juice and within a short time I feel better.

Two years ago I went with my son's Boy Scout troop on a 15-mile hike—just to see if I could do it. My poor feet and legs were hurting so badly by the time I got back to our campsite. I took four ounces of noni juice, crawled inside my sleeping bag and rested in front of the campfire. Within 2 hours all my pain was gone.

I will never underestimate the power of this incredible juice. I will drink my maintenance dose of one to two ounces a day forever!

Skin Infections

There may be nothing more annoying than burning, itchy, swollen, painful skin irritations. Skin problems come in many shapes and sizes. Some people have boils, others eczema. Some have acne, others ulcers. Be sure to add to the list scalp irritations, athlete's foot, and impetigo. The list could go on and on. Whatever the problem, the common link between them all is infection from typically a bacteria, fungus, or even virus.

According to Scott Gerson, M.D., of the Mt. Sinai School of Medicine in New York, the most common and best documented uses of noni address a variety of skin conditions including: wounds, ulcers abscesses, cellulitis, boils, sores, ringworm, bruises, and scalp conditions.

Dr. Gerson has been involved with a research study on a group of patients with eczema. First, it should be noted that eczema can be caused or exacerbated by bacteria. In fact, most experts believe eczema is caused by an abnormality in the immune system. People with eczema release more specialized white blood cells (known as mast cells). Also, the immune systems in people with eczema are often less effective in killing off certain bacteria such as staphylococcus. In his study, Dr. Gerson has found that noni has the ability to "both reduce the amount of histamine and several other allergic substances released from mast cells, and it also has anti-staphylococcal activity."

"In less than three months Synne's skin became like silk!"

Nina Elizabeth Berg relates what happened when her two-year-old with severe psoriasis began using noni juice.

In the spring of 2001, when Synne was two, some small skin rashes appeared on her bottom. During the summer these rashes gradually spread down the inside of her thighs. In August the rashes had exploded, and a dermatologist diagnosed psoriasis. Three treatments from a homeopath did nothing to help. Expensive creams and salves were applied. They alleviated the problem a little, but we finally resorted to cortisone when she began lying awake at nights crying and scratching until her sores bled.

Synne began taking two teaspoons of noni juice twice a day on November 23rd. The next day she was clearly worse, and after another day she became worse than ever. After five days on the juice something dramatic happened. Suddenly she was 70 percent better. All of the thick, red patches on her skin had disappeared. Only the sores where she had been scratching remained, together with some tiny red lumps. But soon our little girl was covered with these lumps.

Many of the lumps festered, and they resembled boils or acne. On December 4th, the twelfth day on the juice, we increased Synne's dose to one tablespoon of noni juice twice a day. After two weeks, another regression occurred. Then her skin cleared again.

January 14th, Synne's dose was increased to one tablespoon three times a day. The next day she had her third regression: redness and an outbreak of more red lumps. By January 19th, she still had the hard, red lumps but they were slightly less red. The dose was increased again to one tablespoon four times a day. By January 22nd Synne's skin was perfectly clear!

By the middle of February, Synne's skin had become like silk and has remained so to this day.

Another researcher who has observed how the ingredients in noni may help skin infections heal more quickly is Dr. Ralph Heinicke. In his book, The Xeronine System, Dr. Heinicke tells of a doctor who used natural components that are also found in noni to treat patients with severe burns. Dr. Klein was a young medical officer turned doctor. After the horror that he saw during the war, he decided to start a general medical practice for the treatment of burns. During his years of research, he developed a burn treatment based on a xeronine-rich bromelain paste that gave results that appeared to be almost miraculous.

He had one particular patient, a young woman who had been trapped in the back seat of a Corvette when the car was rear-ended and burst into flames, who was brought to him with three-fourths of her body extensively burned. The standard hospital prognosis for the future of this patient was one year in the intensive burn ward and then several years of remedial treatment. Even after that she would still be badly scarred.

Dr. Klein started his xeronine-rich bromelain treatment and three months later the woman was well enough to go dancing! Six months later she married in a low-cut dress. These sorts of stories happened again and again during Dr. Klein's practice. He attributed his success to the active ingredients (which Dr. Heinicke later called xeronine) found in the bromelain. Dr. Heinicke reports that noni is the most potent current-day source of xeronine.

"We believe in using natural things to boost our health—noni juice being the top priority."

Sharon Boniek uses noni juice topically to help with a burn.

One time while at our son's home in the mountains of Colorado, I was caring for four little children. We had a huge fire roaring in the wood stove. The two little girls came in from outside, laughing and having fun. One took her boots off, and put her hands on the red-hot stove to brace herself. In an instant both of her hands were horribly burned. I immediately put some noni juice on two napkins, and wrapped her hands in a towel. She still screamed in pain so I put her hands in the ice cold mountain water treated with noni juice. That calmed her. Before she went to bed I put another noni compress on each hand and wrapped them in a towel with a piece of frozen meat. She slept well and was back to her usual self in the morning. Although there were tiny blisters, it could have been so much worse. She has no scars!

Complementary Therapies to Noni

SUPPLEMENTATION

Garlic (Allium Sativum). Garlic has been used for years to treat things such as ear infections, colds, and tuberculosis. It has antibacterial properties that help fight a myriad of infections. Garlic may protect against infectious pathogens by blocking the enzymes that enable the pathogen to enter the tissues of the body.

Gotu Kola (Centella Asiatica). Gotu kola is known as a longevity herb, and it is used widely in India as part of Ayurveda traditional medicine. The red flowered plant grows naturally in swampy areas, and its roots and leaves are used for medicinal purposes such as treating skin disorders.

Grape Seed. Grape seed comes from the tiny seeds of red grapes, and they are a rich source of flavanoids called proanthocyanidins. It has been found to be very helpful with the healing of wounds, bruising, and fragile skin.

Green Tea (Camellia Sinensis). Green tea is derived from the leaves of the tea plant and it is rich in beneficial compounds called catechins. Traditional Chinese medicine has prescribed Green Tea for a strong immune system. It has been shown to help with infections such as tooth decay, digestive infections, as well as respiratory infections.

Licorice Root (Glycyrrhiza Glabra). Licorice root comes from a tall shrub with bluish flowers of the pea family and is found all across Asia and Europe. The root is used medicinally and is one of the most important herbs in traditional Chinese medicine. Licorice root is used for digestive and urinary problems, as well as coughs and sore throats.

Schizandra (Schisandra Chinensis). Schizandra is a woody vine with clusters of red berries that is found in northern and northeastern China and in adjacent regions such as Russia and Korea. Schizandra contains essential oils, acids, and lignans that are believed to help regenerate liver tissue damaged by things like hepatitis. Some studies have shown that schizandra is effective against the bacteria related to lung disorders.

OTHER CONSIDERATIONS

Using noni topically can be accomplished by either applying the juice directly on the skin or by soaking cheese cloth in noni and then applying the cheese cloth to the affected area. Also, noni creams and extracts have been made to make topical use more convenient.

Chapter Summary Points

- Historical data, as well as current research, gives validity to the notion that noni can help fight infection from various sources, particularly by modulating the immune system's production of various anti-infectious agents.

- Noni has been shown to fight various bacteria, viruses, and fungi. For example, scopoletin, a health-promoting agent found in noni, may inhibit the activity of E. coli, commonly associated with recent infectious outbreaks.

- Dr. Scott Gerson has studied the success of noni in patients with eczema, and has found noni to be anti-staphylococcal.

- Dr. Ralph Heinicke attributes the success many have had with treating burns to xeronine found in noni.

Chapter
11
Mental Health

Mental illness has always been around. King Saul in the Bible is said to have had severe depression. During different times in history, society wrongly viewed mental illness as a possession by supernatural forces. In fact, ancient human skulls have been found with large holes in them, a process that was believed to let evil spirits out.

Fortunately, in the classical Greek era, attempts were made to explain physical and psychological phenomenon with more scientific approaches. Those such as Hippocrates and Aristotle insisted that illness (including mental disorders) must be explained on the basis of natural causes, rooted in man's physical structure. However, during the medieval time period, these progressive views were forgotten, and very little advancement was made in better understanding depression and other mental health issues.

Then, at the end of the 1800s, Sigmund Freud's theories arrived on the scene. Freud's work, along with others, pushed toward psychoanalysis as the main and sole treatment for mental illness. This was the "norm" until the 1970s, which brought with them renewed interest in genetic, biochemical, and neuropathological causes of mental health problems. Currently, we have arrived at a combination approach to treating and understanding mental health issues.

Learning the slow and often misguided history of mental health research helps us better understand why there remains even today a sort of "secrecy" surrounding the very common, treatable problem of mental illnesses such as depression and anxiety.

"I had no idea it was going to help, but it did."

Devastated for years from bipolar depression, Tom Corbett tells how noni changed his outlook on life.

About 15 years ago I was diagnosed with bipolar manic-depressive illness. It affected my life so completely for the last three or four years that I couldn't work. I spent most of my day sleeping on the couch. I took numerous antidepressants, and I was even hospitalized. At one point I became suicidal.

Then I got a call from a friend, and he told me about noni juice. Well, I laughed and said, "You're going to tell me this juice is going to do something for me? You don't even know my case history." However, my wife and I went to a convention about noni juice anyway. While there, I asked the keynote speaker, who was a doctor, "Does this product work on someone with severe manic depression?"

He said, "Well, I can't make any promises. I can tell you this product has helped a lot of people." That comment alone opened my heart to the possibilities.

After the convention was over, some friends gave me a bottle of noni. I started by drinking about an ounce and a half. I felt the effects very soon afterwards. I had no idea it was going to help, but it did.

A year has passed. I've not been in the hospital. I have no depression. I take no medication. It's a miraculous thing that happened to me.

Causes and Symptoms

While everyone experiences variations in mood, there are many who suffer from either severe or prolonged depression or anxiety that interferes with the ability to function, feel pleasure, or maintain interest. Depression is a common medical disorder characterized by feelings of sadness, hopelessness, pessimism, restlessness, a change in appetite, problems concentrating or making decisions, and a general loss of interest in life, combined with a sense of reduced emotional well-being. Anxiety is characterized by symptoms such as difficulty sleeping, dizziness, dry mouth, headaches, muscle tension, rapid heartbeat, tingling in extremities, digestive problems, irritability, and withdrawing from others.

Depression and anxiety are problems that originate in the brain. Brain imaging technologies show that in depression neural circuits responsible for the regulation of moods, thinking, sleep, appetite, and behavior fail to function properly. Anxiety is shown to be the effect of the body releasing abnormal amounts of adrenalin and cortisol, which triggers the "flight or fight" response and prepares a person for danger even if there is none. With both conditions, critical neurotransmitters such as serotonin and norepinephrine are off balance.

Vulnerability to these two disorders may result from your genetic make-up combined with specific psychological and environmental factors, such as a loss of a loved one or any stressful change in life patterns. Illnesses such as a heart attack, stroke, or cancer also can cause depressive symptoms.

Unfortunately, difficulties with mental health often go unrecognized or untreated. Each year, an estimated 19 million Americans suffer from depression, making it the most prevalent mental disorder in the country. Not far behind is anxiety. And many times the two go hand-in-hand.

Mental Health
Fact

Four out of every five runaway youths suffer from depression
—*U.S. Select Committee on Children, Youth & Families*

The good news is that most mental health problems respond extremely well to treatment. Those who have the best success typically use a combination treatment. Most people find a combination treatment of conventional medicine, alternative therapies, and professional counseling to be very effective.

As part of that alternative treatment, noni may be very helpful in restoring not only energy to the body, as we talked about in Chapter Seven, but also in regulating the brain's neurotransmitters, such as serotonin. Several prominent researchers, such as Dr. Ralph Heinicke, postulate that noni can enhance the body's utilization of serotonin. Recent years have expanded our knowledge of serotonin and the multiple roles it plays in relieving conditions like depression, anxiety, and sleep dysfunction. Serotonin helps with these conditions because of the role it plays in the brain and nervous system. Dr. Heinicke's extensive research revealing noni's part in the body's production and proper utilization of serotonin provides us with exciting possibilities as to how noni may regulate brain chemical irregularities.

Another important way noni may promote better mental health is through the creation of the alkaloid xeronine in the body. Xeronine production in the body is believed to help explain why noni has spurred reports of better sleep both historically and in modern times. When you sleep, your body is able to produce more serotonin. When you have depression or anxiety, one of the very common symptoms is interrupted sleep. This symptom then feeds the disease by decreasing the one thing you need most…serotonin. If by drinking noni you are able to sleep better, the body can start to replenish its supply of serotonin, which helps you regain overall better mental health.

"Within six weeks I woke up without pain for the first time in years!"

Gloria Schanely, a 44-year-old court interpreter from Lake Placid, Florida, credits noni juice with healing her body of numerous health problems—some dating back as far as 40 years!

Since I can remember, I have suffered with constipation, sinusitis, PMS (mine was pre, present & postmenstrual syndrome), gastritis, depression, arthritis, issues related to viral meningitis, and migraines.

I woke up every morning with pain. If it wasn't my sinusitis, it was my arthritis. If it wasn't my gastritis, it was another migraine. And if any one of these problems were combined with my menstrual cycle, forget it! I would not even be able to get out of bed, much less go to work. I guess the most difficult problems to deal with, were those related to the viral meningitis. I couldn't remember things or people. My brain was foggy and my memory was very poor. I had difficulty with my job and lost several court contracts, etc.

In January of 1999, I read some pretty fascinating stories about people who'd been healed from migraines, gastritis, etc., simply by taking noni juice. I decided to see what noni could do for me, so in February I started taking one ounce in the morning and one ounce in the afternoon. After I finished the first bottle, I upped my dose with another ounce in the afternoon. Within six weeks—March 15th, to be exact—guess what? I woke up without pain for the first time in years! And the positive effects from the noni juice have increased.

My menstrual cycles are better now, and I can function normally throughout them. My sinus condition has totally cleared up, and I don't wake up congested. I am sleeping like a baby, and I don't wake up with gastritis pains any more. I have renewed energy. I am able to eat tomatoes and the other foods I was forced to stay away from. Even milk is fine. Constipation, (something that I've battled since I was a child) is no longer a problem. I have all prescription and over-the-counter pain medications high on my kitchen shelf. I don't need any of them anymore! When I feel a migraine coming on, I just take another ounce of noni juice

The most remarkable thing is that I am thinking straight and I have my confidence back. My thoughts are clear and in order. My brain is balanced, and I have the edge back for my field of work. In court the other day, I was able to raise the judge's eyebrows with my translation skills.

Besides the big changes I've seen with noni, I keep noticing other little things that have improved. My varicose veins don't hurt, and I don't have swelling in my legs anymore. I have long fingernails, my skin tone is beautiful and I have this glow about me. I feel happy, satisfied, and content—feelings I haven't felt in years. I am eager to help others discover the benefits of noni juice!

Alzheimer's Disease

In today's world, more people than ever have memory problems. The most common is Alzheimer's disease. In fact, in the United States the seventh leading cause of death is Alzheimer's disease, and the number of individuals diagnosed with Alzheimer's is doubling every five years. The current annual cost is estimated to be in excess of $60 billion dollars.

Alzheimer's disease is named after Dr. Alois Alzheimer, a German doctor. In 1906, Dr. Alzheimer noticed abnormalities in the brain tissue of a woman who had died of an unusual mental illness. In this woman's brain, he found abnormal clumps (amyloid plaques) and tangled bundles of fibers (neurofibrillary tangles), both of which are now known to be symptoms of Alzheimer's.

Alzheimer's disease starts slowly but has a specific pattern it follows. People with Alzheimer's literally forget routines and habits they have known forever. They experience gradual memory loss, disorientation, personality changes, and an inability to perform basic, everyday tasks. They also experience loss of language, learning, and communication skills. Eventually, a person can forget automatic responses such as how to breathe.

While scientists still do not know the exact cause of Alzheimer's, they do know the risk factors. Age, family history, high blood pressure, high cholesterol, and low levels of the vitamin folate may predispose people to contracting Alzheimer's. Social isolation is another possible cause of cognitive decline. Environmental toxins and previous brain trauma may also predict the occurrence of Alzheimer's disease.

Another recent discovery connected to Alzheimer's is that it is associated with inflammation of the brain cells. This inflammation is believed to be caused by the COX 2 enzyme, the same enzyme that is connected to arthritis and some genetic cancers. Noni juice is a proven COX 2 inhibitor, and it may help those with Alzheimer's in this area.

> **"It's like having a new person in the house!"**
>
> **Ginger Caudill originally got the noni juice for her daughter and herself, but eventually tried it with her sister who'd been diagnosed with schizophrenia and autism. Within three days of taking noni juice her sister showed great progress.**
>
> *My sister, Elizabeth, was diagnosed with autism and schizophrenia more than 20 years ago. She is also retarded. For quite some time she's had a flat effect, probably due to the medication she's on. She has been robotic, and displayed the delayed responses associated with her medications.*
>
> *Three days of one ounce of noni juice twice a day and she was laughing at cartoons on television and interacting with us far more than before. After one week on noni juice she was speaking with inflection in her voice, asking if there was anything she could do for us. It's like having a new person in the house! Her eyes light up and her spirit is finally able to express itself through the physical prison she's been in for so long. Elizabeth is showing remarkable strides, and I credit noni's biochemical effect with these improvements.*

ADHD

Concentration problems in children (and adults) are another area in which noni has been shown to possibly help. Attention Deficit/Hyperactivity Disorder (ADHD) is a type of neurological illness that affects behavior, mood, and learning. Because of the controversy around whether it is or isn't an illness, and the fact that it is being diagnosed in an overwhelming large number of children, this disorder is seeing a lot of attention as of late. Symptoms of ADHD are inattention, hyperactivity, language problems, and impulsive behavior. Some children have the disorder without hyperactivity. Experts say about one child in every classroom has ADHD. Causes are, once again, not certain. However, there does seem to be brain chemistry irregularities and mal-neuro-functioning in children with ADHD. The disorder tends to run in families, according to The National Institute of Mental Health and the American Academy of Pediatrics.

Most children diagnosed with ADHD have impaired neuro-brain-function. This impairment limits the ability to read and utilize language correctly, no matter what language the child may speak. Early and proper reading intervention can improve the reading skills of an estimated 90 percent of those children with ADHD.

In the case of ADHD, noni may be helpful through its ability to modulate the production of some of the chemicals in the brain, (such as serotonin) as well as increase overall cellular health in the brain.

"After four months on noni juice the school was calling my mom, telling her how great I was doing!"

Rients Hettinga, a young boy with ADHD, had problems with concentration and violent outbursts. He fought with his mother daily. Everything changed when he started taking noni juice.

When I was four I had a very hard time communicating. I was withdrawn and moody. When I was six, I was diagnosed with ADHD and put on medication. By the time I was eight, I developed Tourette's-like symptoms. At school I couldn't sit in my desk or concentrate. I was out of control. I started having violent outbursts, breaking another boy's nose and sending a girl to the hospital for stitches. I didn't know why I felt so frustrated inside, but I couldn't help myself.

My Mom and I fought every day about homework and whatever trouble I had gotten into that day. We would both end up crying. I had headaches and was constipated. Every couple of months I became violently ill. When I heard about noni juice I started taking three ounces a day, and within two months I was off my ADHD medication. After four months on noni juice the school was calling my mom, telling her how great I was doing!

It has been one year since I started taking noni juice. I am a different boy. I feel happy, and I have friends. My mom and I no longer fight. Instead we can communicate and have loving conversations. Now I tell my mom about other kids that need help from noni juice. I want them to be happy too. I love my noni!

Noni as a Detoxifier

One of the common links to all mental health issues is the role pollution and modern chemicals play in the cause of mental illness. While there is much talk of this connection, it has been very hard to prove. Nonetheless, many doctors are now telling their patients of the benefits of detoxifying the body in order to prevent chemical build up that may eventually cause cellular damage in the brain.

In his book *Noni, Healing, and You,* Dr. Scott Gerson explains that toxic substances are delivered to the liver through the blood. The liver, if it gets too full, will signal to the body that it can no longer keep up with the amount of toxins it is receiving by symptoms such as chronic fatigue, constipation, acne, psoriasis, depression, anxiety, confusion, and even learning disabilities. It is reported that as much as 30 percent of the U.S. population suffers from toxicity.

During his doctoral work, Dr. Gerson focused on the effect of Ayurvedic massage therapies to reduce toxicity. Two years into the study, he decided to add noni juice to the treatment. What he found was that noni, when combined with Ayurvedic massage techniques, increased the rate of liver detoxification by more than 50 percent. He believes why noni is effective in detoxification is because it may help prevent the depletion of a natural substance called glutathione, a chemical critical for the correct detoxification of the liver.

"Within three days she was able to focus better in school and at home."

Julie Lowe, a mother from Kennett, Missouri, was afraid of repeating the ADHD experience with another child. She and her husband are so pleased with the difference noni juice has made in their daughter's life.

When my 26-year-old son was younger we suffered all kinds of grief as he struggled with ADHD. When my 10-year old daughter, Mary Elizabeth, began to exhibit the same symptoms, I wasn't interested in repeating the experience. I started her on a morning dose of one ounce of noni juice. Within three days she was able to focus better in school and at home. She was not as hyper or emotional. She already had lots of energy, but the noni juice seemed to even out her moods so she didn't burn out as easily. When she fell asleep, she slept more soundly. Her allergies improved tremendously, as well.

Mary Elizabeth is a gymnast, competing with the United States Gymnastics Team in Blytheville, Arkansas. One evening after a strenuous workout, she complained of leg-muscle pain. She had worked out more than usual on the bars and had small, vein-break looking bruises on the back of her leg. The soreness from intense workouts usually lasts a couple of days, but she'd never had the bruising before. So in addition to the noni juice therapy I applied the noni Skin Supplement to the bruises and leg muscles. The next morning she had no muscle pain, and the bruising was noticeably lighter. That evening the bruising and muscle pain were completely gone.

I accidentally ran out of noni juice after she had been taking it for a week, so she was without it for three or four days. She came home from gym practice one evening and dramatically asked when the noni juice would arrive—she couldn't wait! She noticed she didn't have the same energy she had been having with the noni juice. I noticed she was losing focus rapidly, becoming forgetful and scattered.

Now she takes one ounce of noni juice in the morning and one ounce in the evening. Her behavior is better, and she is doing better in school again. And she has more energy for her workouts. My husband and I are very happy she is back on noni juice. It has made a huge difference in all of our lives.

Complementary Therapies to Noni

DIET/NUTRITION RECOMMENDATIONS

Eating a diet high in complex carbohydrates and low in fats and refined sugar may help bring stability to brain chemical imbalances. Additionally, Omega-3 fatty acids are widely believed to be effective in boosting serotonin levels and in helping with mental health problems. Omega-3 is found in fish such as salmon. Also, avoiding caffeine and alcohol is strongly recommended.

SUPPLEMENTATION

Damiana (Turnera Aphrodisiaca). Damiana contains terpenes, beta-sitoserol, arbutin, alkaloids, and various aromatic oils that may help alleviate anxiety and promote a sense of well-being.

DHEA (Dehydroepiandrosterone). DHEA is a hormone produced by the adrenal glands concerned with biological activity throughout the body and brain. DHEA production, for both men and women, dramatically decreases with age starting at approximately age 25. By the time people reach age 75, DHEA production drops to approximately 95 percent of what it was at age 25. By increasing DHEA levels, you may increase feelings of well-being, improve sleep, have more energy, and better handle stress.

Ginkgo Biloba. Ginkgo biloba is an ancient tree found in China and Japan that has been around for more than 200 million years. Ginkgo biloba is believed to increase blood flow and oxygen to the brain to help alleviate memory-related problems.

Ginseng. Ginseng has been used for more than 5,000 years. It is used in traditional Chinese medicine as a preventative tonic to stimulate the entire body to overcome stress, fatigue, and weakness. Some strains of Ginseng have shown to help produce endorphins, which are natural chemicals in the body that make people feel good.

Guarana (Paullinia Cupana). The substance guaranine in guarana has traces of alkaloids like theophylline and theobromine (which are found in chocolate and cocoa) that work as a stimulant to increase mental and physical alertness and performance.

Oats (Avena Sativa). Oats help strengthen the nervous system when one is under stress. They have also been shown to calm down performance anxiety. Oats are rich in silicon, manganese, zinc, calcium, phosphorus and Vitamins A, B1, B2, and E.

SAM-e (s-adenosylmethiodine.) SAM-e is produced from a yeast derivative and was introduced to the United States in 1999. It is a substance found naturally in the body that is believed to fuel dozens of biochemical reactions and is backed by many studies done in Europe. It is believed to work by enhancing the action of two mood-regulating brain chemicals—serotonin and dopamine.

St. John's Wort (Hypericum perforatum). St. John's Wort has a 2,400-year history of safe and effective usage in folk, herbal, and ancient medicine. Hypericum was prescribed as medicine by Hippocrates himself. Studies indicate that Hypericum perforatum may be an effective antidepressant with far fewer side effects than prescription medication.

Valerian Root. Valerian has been used as a sleep aid for more than 1,000 years. It is believed to help relax the central nervous system, promote feelings of calm, decrease levels of anxiety and stress, and enhance sleep. Unlike prescription sleep aids, valerian is not known to cause morning grogginess and is non-addictive.

OTHER CONSIDERATIONS

Psychotherapy. In one form of psychotherapy called cognitive behavioral therapy, patients learn coping strategies to counteract the obsessive thoughts of failure, inadequacy, and pervasive gloom that accompany depression and anxiety. In a 2002 study conducted at Vanderbilt University in Nashville and the University of Pennsylvania, cognitive behavioral therapy was compared to the use of prescription medication for moderate-to-severe depression. Results showed the medicated group got better more quickly, but after about four months both groups had an equal percentage who had improved. After an additional year, the cognitive therapy patients fared much better. In fact, 75 percent of them remained symptom-free, compared with 60 percent of patients on medication, and 19 percent on a placebo.

Light therapy. This treatment has been used for a while to treat seasonal affective disorder, a type of depression that afflicts about one in ten people who live in places with short winter days and extended darkness. Current studies, however, indicate that being bathed with at least 30 minutes a day in bright artificial light may be as effective as an antidepressant at any time of the year. In a 2002 study of 16 pregnant women with major depression, one hour of light therapy improved their symptoms by 49 percent after three weeks, a response rate comparable to prescription antidepressants.

Exercise. Numerous studies have shown exercise to be an excellent antidote for mild-to-moderate depression. Duke researchers studied the effects of exercise on 156 volunteers older than age 50 who were diagnosed with depression. After 16 weeks, those on the exercise treatment had the same level of improvement as those on prescription medication, although those who took antidepressants got faster relief from their symptoms. However, a follow-up study 10 months later found the exercise group had a significantly lower relapse rate for depression than those on medication.

Other therapies for better mental health include acupuncture, yoga, massage therapy, and relaxation techniques.

Anyone with a serious mental-health problem should always consult his or her doctor before changing any treatment.

Chapter Summary Points

- Depression and anxiety are problems that originate in the brain.

- Vulnerability to mental-health problems may result from genetic makeup combined with specific psychological and environmental factors, such as a loss of a loved one or any stressful change in life patterns. Illnesses such as a heart attack, stroke, or cancer also can cause depressive symptoms.

- Noni may be helpful in restoring energy to the body, and in helping regulate the brain's neurotransmitters, such as serotonin. Several prominent researchers, such as Dr. Ralph Heinicke, postulate that noni can enhance the body's utilization of serotonin.

- Concentration and memory problems such as ADHD and Alheimer's may also respond positively to noni. Noni inhibits the COX 2 enzyme, which has been shown to be involved with brain cell inflammation in Alzheimer's.

- Many feel toxicity is linked to mental-health problems. Dr. Scott Gerson found that noni, when combined with Ayurvedic massage techniques, increased the rate of liver detoxification by more than 50 percent. He believes why noni is effective in detoxification is because it may help prevent the depletion of a natural substance called glutathione.

Weight Control

How many people do you know who have high blood pressure, diabetes, elevated cholesterol, depression, heart disease, or even cancer? Have you ever wondered if all these disease had one thing in common? Well, they do. One of the common links to all these diseases (and about 55 others) is obesity.

Obesity is killing us—literally. In fact, it is the second leading preventable cause of death in the United States, right behind tobacco use. Nearly one-third of all adults are now classified as obese, according to data from the 1999-2000 National Health and Nutrition Examination Survey published in the *Journal of the American Medical Association.* Another one-third of Americans are overweight. That means two out of three Americans is at major risk for disease. So, if there are three people in a room, which person are you?

A Few of the Health Conditions Linked to Weight

- cancer
- chronic fatigue
- depression
- diabetes
- heart disease
- high blood pressure
- lowered resistance to infection
- stroke

Poor food choices, sedentary lifestyles, and technological advances are all responsible for adding to our weight problem. However, there still remains some mystery as to why some people gain a lot of weight, and others don't. Yes, diet and exercise have something to do with it, but so do genetics and body type. There are biological factors at play. Recent studies show that obese people take longer to feel full, even if they eat the same amount of food as someone of normal weight. One study by Yijun Liu, Ph.D. at the University of Florida, closely studied 10 obese people and 20 people of normal weight and how their brains interpreted food intake.

In this study, researchers gave the study participants glucose transmitted through an IV. Then each subject received 350 MRI scans. Signals in the obese subjects' brains were weaker and significantly delayed by four to nine minutes, showing that their bodies were receiving the "I'm full" signal from their brains a lot slower than someone of normal weight.

"Even my kids have noticed the difference!"

Terri Kosinski, a 55-year-old mother using noni juice to help with weight loss, shares her success:

To date, I have lost 33 pounds and 11 inches all over my body. I drink my noni one half-hour before I eat, and then I sip more after each meal. I believe the noni has helped me to digest my food better. I eat a low-carb diet and I have included a walking program into my daily routine.

Family and friends tell me I look thinner. Even my kids have noticed the difference! I have another 20 pounds to lose, and I know it is possible. Noni juice has changed my life in so many ways. Thanks to noni juice, I love the way I look and feel!

Other studies using twins have shown a genetic biological cause to weight gain. Studies about adopted children who have similarities in body mass to their biological parents not to their adoptive parents again show there are genetic tendencies for obesity. Some reasons for these genetic tendencies focus on the body's endocrine system, or the system that makes our hormones. For example, the hormone ghreline is produced in the stomach and small intestine, and it is the only natural appetite stimulant to be made outside the brain. People given shots of ghreline eat 30 percent more than normal. So it's possible that too much naturally made ghreline contributes to weight gain.

Another hormone known as peptide YY3-36, or PYY, is released in the body in response to food. It circulates to the brain where it decreases our urge to eat. If our body doesn't make enough PYY, we will never know we are full.

Because of this "biological" tendency to be overweight, many people who have already changed both their diets and their lifestyles are looking for an added boost to help them in their weight loss goals. That may be the reason many are turning to a natural food supplement like noni. Those drinking noni have reported having more energy, a more positive outlook on life, and better overall nutrition. This third point is no small matter. Good nutrition is overlooked with people wanting to lose weight. Sadly, we can be overweight and poorly nourished at the same time.
A few of the consequences from unhealthy dieting include:

- Decreased cardiac output
- Decreased cognition (thinking)
- Difficulty in fighting infections
- Increased dementia and delirium
- Increased falls and hip fractures
- Increased peripheral edema
- Increased risk of infections
- Poor wound healing
- Weakness and fatigue

"It took only two weeks to lose the 18 pounds I've been struggling to get off for 14 months!"

A noni protein drink is an excellent adaptogen, as this couple found out.

Since David's illness two years ago, I have been making him a noni protein shake daily. Two weeks ago I decided to start drinking them too. Right away my energy picked up and the evening binges stopped. I had to try to remember to eat at least once a day. Within a few days I noticed my clothes were fitting better. It took only two weeks to lose the 18 pounds I'd been struggling to get off for 14 months! And that was without exercise or any special dieting. Yippeee!

I make shakes by the quart and keep them refrigerated so they're ready any time.

My recipe for a one-quart shake is:
1 cup water, 2 ounces of noni juice, four scoops of a noni-based protein drink, three big scoops of "no sugar added" chocolate ice cream, 1 teaspoon sugar or other sweetener.

Blend all ingredients and pour into a quart container. Add water to fill the bottle and shake well. Keep refrigerated and shake well before pouring yourself a delicious drink.

Sometimes I use "no sugar added" vanilla ice cream and fresh strawberries, blueberries, or peaches.

David has gained a few pounds like he needed, and I have lost weight. Is this stuff great or what? I guess that's what it means when they say noni is an adaptogen.

Losing Pounds with Noni

Most of my life as a retired endocrinologist who specialized in metabolism has been spent studying weight loss. For 30 years I saw on average 1,000 patients yearly strictly for obesity/metabolism problems. That translates into about 30,000 obesity patients during my medical career. On average each patient lost about 20 pounds of fat. That means during my career I saw my patients lose approximately three hundred tons of fat from their bodies. And yes, they did this all without noni juice since noni was not available in the United States when I was practicing.

However, we now know much more about weight loss than we did back then. We also know more about how natural substances work in the body as adaptogens and natural modulators. Yes, you can lose weight without noni. However, by incorporating noni into your diet you may find, as many others have done, that your weight loss is easier to accomplish and more effective than without noni.

I have always believed that good health and a healthy weight begin with good nutrition, regular exercise, and a positive attitude about life. However, since so many modern foods we ingest are so depleted of vitamins and nutrients, I believe we must take a closer look at nutritional food supplements like noni for help.

Noni helps with weight loss through various means. First of all, with the increased energy that people report after drinking noni juice, a person is more apt to feel like he or she has the strength to exercise. Another way in which noni may play an important role in weight loss is through its ability to promote the creation of xeronine in the body. Xeronine is the cellular-enhancing alkaloid that is in short demand in the body. Another way in which noni may encourage weight loss is by its powerful antioxidant action. Noni also has been reported by thousands to promote better sleep, and better sleeping habits have been recently linked by scientists to a healthy metabolism.

Research released in *Endocrine Today* shows that without enough sleep, the body's metabolism may decrease, making it more difficult for people to lose or maintain weight. Lack of sleep decreases the body's production of the growth hormone, which is an important hormone in maintaining weight. On average, we need about eight hours of sleep a night. According to a recent survey by the National Sleep Foundation, only 30 percent of adults in the United Stated report getting eight or more hours of sleep per weeknights.

Another large part of weight gain is from what is called the snowball effect. Once you gain a little weight, that weight impacts your body, making you more tired, more lethargic, and worn out. So you don't or can't do anything about the little bit of weight you've gained, and doing nothing eventually leads to more weight gain. The snowball grows from there. When you drink noni juice, you are putting a damper in the snowball's descent. You give your body the extra boost it needs to start attacking the weight.

"Finally, I am high-school skinny again!"

Noni products gave Jenna Robinson her life back. She has no more problems with arthritis, migraines, acid reflux or high cholesterol. She's also back to her dream weight.

I was introduced to noni juice about three years ago. I suffered with arthritis, migraine headaches, acid reflux and high cholesterol. After drinking noni juice for just a few short weeks I no longer suffered pain from any of those health problems. And to top it off, I lost 40 pounds in just six months using a noni-based weight-loss program called the Tahiti Trim. Finally, I am high school skinny again!

Another reason for using noni for weight loss is because of its ability to fight free-radical damage through its antioxidant action. Included in the 150 nutraceuticals (natural food components) found in noni are some of the most powerful antioxidants known such as proanthocyanadins, anthocyanidins, vitamin C, and many others. In a test for antioxidant activity, noni scored higher than some of the better-known antioxidants of the day.

Antioxidants are extremely important in weight loss because they help restore health on a cellular level. When the body's cells don't function at 100 percent, the body may slip into survival mode. In survival mode, the body may hold on to weight for what it believes may be upcoming "hard times." The body believes if things are bad, they could even get worse, and therefore it prepares itself for a long winter, like a bear going into hibernation.

"I found that the inches melted away and gave shape to my body."

Priscilla Salazar Martínez got more than she expected when she started the noni weight loss program-better overall health and a new body shape!

In October of 1996, I was introduced to noni juice. At the time I weighed more than I had during any of my four pregnancies. I began the noni weight-loss program so I could lose weight in a healthy way. Each morning I take an ounce of noni juice and swish it in my mouth for 30 seconds before swallowing it. I drink 2 glasses of water and nothing more for the next 30 minutes. This gives the noni juice time to work its magic.

Almost immediately I experienced more energy and no more insomnia. After a month or so I noticed joint aches and pains were gone.

Inches started to melt away. In the first few months of using this program, my body began to change shape. Throughout the entire program I only lost 20 pounds. I had wanted to lose more, but I found that the inches that melted away gave new shape to my body structure. I went down eight sizes. The amazing thing to me is that my priorities have changed. Greater than the weight and inches lost is the fact that my overall health has improved so drastically. Better overall health has truly been the most wonderful benefit to using noni juice.

Complementary Therapies to Noni

DIET/NUTRITION RECOMMENDATIONS

There are literally hundreds of diets to choose from. Since this is not a diet book, feel free to choose a moderate, sensible diet that you feel you can "stick to." Just make sure the diet includes things such as eating high-complex-carbohydrates, low-saturated fat, and lots of fiber. It should also include plenty of raw vegetables, fruits, and vegetable juices. Eat frequent, smaller meals throughout the day. This can help reduce the need for unhealthy snacking, and it keeps a more normal blood-glucose level.

Any weight-loss diet should tell you to avoid simple carbohydrates. This applies especially to foods high in refined flour and sugar. In addition, more and more experts are finding that people wanting to lose weight should eat a balance of carbohydrates and healthy protein from sources such as grains, legumes, low-fat dairy products, fish, and poultry.

SUPPLEMENTATION

Bilberry, ginkgo, pycnogenol and hawthorn: These all reportedly help protect the arteries, preventing arteriosclerosis, and slow the development of vascular problems common to diabetics, particularly in the eyes and extremities (hands, toes, fingers, etc.)

Chrominum picolinate. Chromium is a naturally occurring mineral. Small amounts of chromium are found in everyday foods like meat, poultry, fish, and whole-grain breads. When foods are processed, however, the natural chromium is lost. Chromium picolinate is simply a nutritional supplement that has combined chromium with picolinic acid to help the body absorb the chromium. This supplement helps to keep an optimal level of insulin in the body. It has been reported to help with a number of different conditions, the most common of which is weight loss.

Digestive enzymes. Because the pancreas also produces other substances that contribute to the proper digestion of food, taking digestive enzyme supplements can relieve stress on the body's digestive system.

Essential fatty acids. Because the body is inhibited in its ability to metabolize EFAs, fatty acids such as gamma linolenic acid (GLA) and eicosapentaenoic acid (EPA) are good supplementation investments.

Fiber supplements. Even though improvements in diet can provide the added benefits of more dietary fiber, it is often helpful to also add a fiber supplement to one's diet. Fiber helps maintain a more even blood-sugar level for extended periods during the day.

Fiber. Fiber has a long list of useful functions in the body, especially functions that relate to weight control. For example, foods high in fiber usually require more chewing, which may help with the actual amount of food eaten. Once in the stomach, fiber feels bulky and this helps the stomach to feel full, thereby helping with appetite suppression. Fiber also attracts water to the digestive tract, which softens stools and prevents constipation. Regular elimination helps with maintaining body balance.

Garcinia cambogia. Garcinia cambogia is a fruit with a distinctive sour flavor that is used in Indian cooking. In more recent years, one of the compounds within the fruit called Hydroxycitric acid (HCA) has been shown to be an appetite suppressant. Studies show HCA can reduce the conversion of carbohydrates into stored fat by slowing down or even stopping a certain enzyme called citrate lyase which is responsible for making new fat cells. HCA also may breakdown fat in the liver and in the fat cells.

L-carnitine. L-carnitine is a substance made in the body from the two amino acids called lysine and methionine. It can also be found in dairy products. L-carnitine carries fatty acids into the cells' mitochondria where it is needed to help release energy from fat. Not only is L-carnitine linked to weight control in the body, but it is also linked to healthy heart function, improved lungs, and a myriad of other functions.

L-glutamine and taurine. These amino acids help the body reduce sugar cravings, improve its ability to produce insulin, and enhance fat utilization.

Vitamin B12 (cobalamin). This vitamin is important in the body because it plays a role in the growth, development, and production of blood cells. It also impacts the functions of the nervous system. It also dictates how the body uses carbohydrates, an important function when it comes to weight loss.

Vitamin B6 (pyridoxine). This vitamin is very useful in weight loss. Vitamin B-6 plays the role of a coenzyme that supports amino acid metabolism. It controls the absorption, metabolism, and conversion of amino acids into neurotransmitters, antibodies, digestive enzymes, muscles, and tissues in the body. It also has an effect on protein, carbohydrate, and fat metabolism. Women in particular might be deficient in B6 because of some of the products they have used. For example, contraceptives negatively affect the body's levels of B6 as well as the use of antidepressants. Other factors that may lead to lower levels of B6 are poor absorption in the gastrointestinal tract, use of antibiotics, and eating only food high in protein.

Zinc, vanadium, manganese, and magnesium. All of these minerals are known to be involved in the body's maintenance of proper blood-sugar levels.

OTHER CONSIDERATIONS

Have a weight loss plan. The following four points are what I consider to be essential strategies for losing weight:

1. Clearly identify your motivating factors.
2. Develop a realistic plan using incremental goals.
3. Put in place tools you will use to reach your goals.
4. Get scientific information from the experts. Don't succumb to fad diets.

Exercise. This goes hand-in-hand with weight management. Exercise can help fight the various forms of heart disease, decrease high blood pressure, lower blood-sugar levels and cholesterol levels, and improve circulation.

Chapter Summary Points

- Obesity is the second leading preventable cause of death in the United States, right behind tobacco use.

- Nearly one-third of all adults are now classified as obese. Another one-third of Americans are overweight.

- Poor food choices, sedentary lifestyles, technological advances, genetics, and body type are all responsible for adding to our weight problem. There are also various biological factors at play.

- Combined with eating right and better exercise, noni may help in an overall weight loss plan. It may help through cellular regeneration, increasing levels of antioxidants, boosting energy, promoting restful sleep, and helping with a positive mental outlook.

SECTION III

Noni's
Proven Track
Record

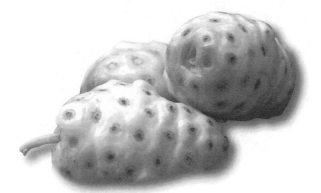

13

Noni—A Safe Player

Imagine yourself sitting on the edge of your couch, watching your favorite basketball team play. Your team is behind only one point with five seconds left in the game. Then, the star player for your team is fouled and you breathe a sigh of relief. Why? Because you know that player has a track record of shooting 90 percent from the free throw line. He is a safe player. His past performance has proven so. You know the game is as good as in the bag.

That is the way I like to look at noni juice. Noni juice is a safe player. Its past 2,000 years of traditional use has shown us that as well as modern testing in a laboratory. Noni has proven itself to thousands, even millions of individuals, through its consistent, safe, productive results.

So much has been said in the media and medical community about the safety, or non-safety, of herbs and natural food supplements. When it comes to noni, specifically TAHITIAN NONI® Juice, put your mind at rest. TAHITIAN NONI® Juice has been tested to see if it contains any of more than 300 different toxins. Every test has come up negative. The juice itself goes through a thermal pasteurization that keeps it safe while allowing the special compounds within the juice to remain active.

Europe's Novel Food Act Committee (much like the U.S. government's FDA) approved noni for sale as a novel food in Europe. It concluded, "There were no indications of adverse effects from laboratory animal studies on subacute and subchronic toxicity, genotoxicity, and allergenic-ity" from noni juice.

Other studies have observed animals and humans consuming up to seven bottles of noni juice a day with no adverse reaction. Of course, there may be some people or animals (and statistically speaking the chance is quite low) who are allergic to some of the ingredients in noni.

Of course, no food product can ever honestly claim that it is non-aller-genic to 100 percent of the population. That is simply impossible. In some cases, minor allergic symptoms to noni may occur. This would include things such as belching, gas, mild transient diarrhea, or a slight rash or itching. If this is the case, reduce the amount of noni consumed until the undesired symptoms disappear. If these symptoms persist, stop drinking noni juice. In the case of a major allergic reaction (persistent diarrhea, hives, swelling, or difficulty in swallowing or breathing) stop drinking noni immediately. When all the symptoms disappear you may try drinking noni again at half the amount. If possible, slowly build back up to the more helpful amount. If any symptoms reappear, stop drinking noni juice. In both cases, notify your health professional and follow his or her advice.

In 2000, some professors at Purdue University published a report clam-ing that noni juice may have been the cause for one man's hyperkalemia, or kidney problems. These researchers claimed that noni contained hid-den amounts of potassium. Since then, tests have shown that TAHITIAN NONI® Juice has less than half the potassium level found in one ounce of orange juice or one ounce of tomato juice. This was documented by the U.S. Department of Agriculture Nutrient Data Laboratory. Therefore, if you are on a low-potassium diet, use the juice as you would these other juice sources.

While collecting my survey data, I have not seen any documented nega-tive reports of using TAHITIAN NONI® Juice for even pregnant and lactating women, children, and the elderly. A few people have reported allergies, hypersensitivities, and other minor problems.

The U.S. Food and Drug Administration and the Department of Agriculture have a list, called the GRAS list, which records plants that have no known harmful ingredients in them. The GRAS list also shows the types of plants that from extended use by a large number of people have proven themselves to be safe for humans for the general population. Noni has been officially designated as a safe plant on this list.

Success with Noni

One of the most convincing aspects for me to drink noni juice is the large number of success stories I personally have received from people who drink noni. I have tried to share as many of these stories as I could throughout this book. As I look back on my research with noni, I am struck by the number of people who are living happier, healthier lives because of this natural gift from Mother Nature. This strange, small, bumpy fruit truly has been the "health solution" for which so many of us have been searching.

"*The vet is testing noni juice on some of his other patients!*"

Deborah Harr, a pet owner from Salt Lake City, Utah, nursed a very sick Labrador back to health with the help of noni juice. Now she has a new best friend!

I have two dogs, two cats, one Iguana, and several injured birds that we are trying to nurse back to health for release. All of our pets drink noni juice every day! Suzie Q, our Labrador, came to us from the local dog pound. She was as thin as could be and very lethargic. Every time we fed her, she would nearly swallow the whole bowl without taking a breath, but she couldn't keep anything down. After doing some tests on her the vet said we would be lucky if she survived the month due to extreme malnutrition. She was on a special diet for six months. Once she was back to a durable health we began bathing her with a special shampoo and applying special cream to her skin to help clear up her bald patches. All the attention did her little good. We couldn't find a permanent home for Suzy Q because she had so many special needs.

My family drinks noni juice as a nutritional supplement, and I'd read about giving noni juice to pets. Nothing else seemed to be working, so we decided to try noni juice with Suzy Q. We dabbed it on her bald patches with a cotton ball, and put one teaspoon in her water bowl each day. At the end of the month, her bald patches were clearing up and she wasn't scratching them. We gradually increased her dose to one ounce a day. No more special shampoos, no more ointments, and no other supplements. It truly has been an amazing change in our Suzie Q! After three months of one ounce of noni juice a day, she is acting like she never had a problem in the world. She plays, jumps, and goes with me when I jog. No more bald patches and no signs that they ever plagued her. She is beautiful now, and her coat is so shiny. She doesn't like the taste of noni juice, so I have to give it to her when she is really thirsty. The other animals take it just fine, including the Iguana. The vet was shocked to see the change in Suzie Q's health. He's even testing noni juice on some of his other patients. We have fallen in love with our Susie Q and are no longer searching for a home for her—she stole our hearts!

"It is not everyday that you see a miracle."

Terri Kosinski tells of her rapid recovery from a broken foot.

I broke my left foot in November. I had a cast put on and was told that I had to wear it for six weeks. My muscles were hurting so bad in the cast for the past few weeks, and I had constant cramps in the calf muscle as well as under the toes.

Since this happened, I have been drinking about 8 ounces or more of noni everyday. On Monday morning I woke up in so much pain from the cramping of the muscles. I called the doctor and he said to come in right away and he would take some more x-rays. He was so amazed. He said, "This is a real miracle. It is healed." He was amazed I had no inflammation or swelling at all.

He wanted to know if I was taking the anti-inflammatory medicine he prescribed for me. This was an open door for me to tell him about noni. He was familiar with the noni, and he said he had other patients who have used it for broken bones and inflammation also.

I told him, "It is not every day that you see a miracle."

"It has already started to heal."

Emily uses a noni-based lip balm for lots of things besides just her lips.

We live in an area where the fire ants are everywhere. When they bothered me in the past it took a day or two for the sting to stop hurting. The other day I got stung several times on the top of my foot. I went in the house to find something to stop the pain, and I found a *noni-based lip balm. I rubbed some on the affected area and went back out to work. That night when I took my shower I couldn't even see where the ants had stung. HOORAY! If you've ever been stung by a fire ant you know what I mean.*

Just a couple of days ago, while I was helping my husband build a new deck, a board fell and gouged the back of my leg. I got the bleeding stopped and went to put a bandage on it, but first I smeared the noni lip balm on it. There is no soreness, and it's already started to heal.

"The doctor said she wouldn't believe the surgery had been done had she not done it herself. We believe noni juice helped him heal faster."

Betty and Neil Comfort have two great healing stories. One for Neil, and one for their dog, Kana.

Neil recently had eye surgery, and during the follow up appointment, three days after surgery, the doctor was amazed at his recovery. She said she wouldn't believe the surgery been done had she not done it herself. We believe noni juice helped him heal faster. He doubled his noni intake a week before and after surgery.

Our dog Kana fell down the stairs and tore a ligament in her hind leg. The vet said the leg would never heal without medical attention. He suggested a $2,500 surgery. Neil and I decided to try noni juice instead.

We started giving Kana one ounce of noni per day along with some other supplements. After several months her limping subsided, and after eight months she was walking and running completely normal-

ly. We took Kana back to the vet and he was amazed at the results. He said she no longer needed the surgery because the knee joint was back to normal. We were very thankful we used the noni therapy instead of the surgery. It would have been miserable for Kana and a huge expense for us!

"After using noni juice for only four months, my allergies were gone!"

Stig Oftedal, a CEO, had severe allergies for 20 years, and is now allergy free—thanks to noni juice.

I had severe allergies after moving to eastern Washington in 1983. In September 2002, I began using noni juice. For the first time in my adult life I was able to stop drinking coffee without experiencing any headaches. Four months later, my allergies were gone. I have not used medication or medical assistance to relieve these symptoms— only noni juice.

It's wonderful to have such a great product to share with friends and business associates!

"After only one application of the noni cream she stopped attacking her incision, and never bothered it again."

Meria Heller, an animal lover, used noni on her 'best friend' with great results.

I got a little Bichon from an animal shelter. She's a beauty! I brought her home right after she was spayed. When I got her home I put a *teaspoon of noni in her mouth right away. Instead of putting a collar on her to keep her from scratching at her incision, I put some noni-based lotion on it. After only one application of the noni she stopped attacking her incision, and never bothered it again.*

Today is her third day home, and thanks to noni juice, she is like a bouncing baby. She has no evidence of pain. She had a messy blob of mucus running from her eye that they were putting drops in. Knowing what noni did for my eye problem, I tried it on hers. The noni juice cleared it up in three days. Noni juice works miracles!

"There is nothing like noni juice for rejuvenating the body. It's great for cleansing the system and the blood."

The Boniek couple went on a noni fast. The wife records the results they enjoyed.

My husband, Elmer, and I decided go on a noni fast. He is 74 and I am 64. We are both in reasonably good health, but he started experiencing some shortness of breath, insomnia and fatigue. We had been using noni juice for four years with great success, so we were excited to see what a noni fast would do. Besides, my husband had gained an enormous amount of weight in his middle. He seemed bloated and couldn't get his pants buttoned. He was showing symptoms of other health issues, as well. This seemed like the perfect time to get serious.

We averaged six to eight noni cocktails the first few days. We did not feel deprived of food. If we felt hungry we sipped another noni cocktail, and that did the trick. The results were absolutely astounding!

Even without food our energy levels were much higher. My husband had trouble getting in as many noni cocktails as I did, because he was so busy. He used to take a nap at eight in the evening and then go to bed around nine. On the noni fast he was still up and working at midnight! We slept well and woke refreshed. (Maybe because my husband's insomnia was gone!) It was definitely a plus for me, not having to cook for five days. It gave me more time to work, with all the energy I had.

By the fourth day of the fast I had lost over seven pounds and Elmer more than fifteen. We decided to do a break-fast combining the noni cocktails with citrus fruit. We noticed some rejuvenation benefits: clearer minds, cleaner feeling inside, and even more energy. Day six we ate fruit and sipped noni cocktails all day and for dinner enjoyed our first meal: a nice salad without dressing. Before bedtime I had two ounces of noni juice with a drink of water.

Sunday was the real test. My husband is a pastor, and I play for our services. Would we be able to get through this morning after a week of fasting? We felt wonderful, strong, energetic, and clear headed. I weighed myself at the end of the day, and I had lost another three pounds. That Sunday my husband looked good (with pants buttoned this time) in his preaching suit!

Our noni fast brought another big surprise. I have suffered with an itchy eyelid for years. Nothing seemed to clear it up. I used to put an ointment on it every night or it would hurt in the morning. I forgot the ointment this past week while we were on the fast, and there was no itchy eyelid!

References

A. Hirazumi, E. Furusawa, S.C. Choud, and Y. Hokama, "Anti-cancer Activity of Morinda citrifolia (Noni) on Intraperitoneally Implanted Lewis Lung Carcinoma in Syngenic Mice," *Proc. West Pharmacol. Soc.* Vol. 376, 1994.

Abbott, I.A., and C. Shimazu. "The Geographic Origin of the Plants most Commonly Used for Medicine by Hawaiians." *Journal of Ethnopharmacology* 14 (1985): 213-22.

Ancolio C, Azas N, Mahiou V, Ollivier E, Di Giorgio C, Keita A, Timon-David P, Balansard G. "Antimalarial activity of extracts and alkaloids isolated from six plants used in traditional medicine in Mali and Sao Tome." *Phytother Res.* 2002 Nov;16(7):646-9.

Bardon S, Picard K, and Martel P. "Monoterpenes inhibit cell growth, cell cycle progression, and cyclin D1 gene expression in human breast cancer cell lines." *Nutr Cancer*, 1998; 32(1), pp. 1-7.

Blakeslee, S. "Surprise Discovery: Hemoglobin Has Bigger Role." *The New York Times*, March 21, 1996: A1-22.

Block, G. "Epidemiologic evidence regarding vitamin C and cancer." *American Journal of Clinical Nutrition* 54 (1991): 1310S-14S.

British Medical Journal ,July 8, 2000;321:88-92.

Burkill, I.H. *A Dictionary of the Economic Products of the Malay Peninsula.* 2 (1966): 1518.

Bushnell, O.A., et al. "The Antibacterial Properties of Some Plants Found in Hawaii." *Pacific Science* 4 (1950): 167-83.

Chafique Younos, Alain Rolland, Jacques Fleurentin, Marie-Claire Lanhers, Rene Misslin, and Francois Mortier, "Analgesic and Behavioural Effects of Morinda citrifolia," *Planta Med*, Vol. 56, 1990.

Cheema-Dhadli S., Harlperin M.L., Leznoff C.C. "Inhibition of enzymes which interact with citrate by hydroxycitrate and 1,2,3,-tricarboxybenzene." *Eur J Biochem* 1973; 38:98–102.

Chronic Fatigue and Immune Dysfunction Association of America. *The CFIDS Chronicle* July/August, 1999.

"COX 2 Shows Up in Stomach Cancers." *Science News*, August 18, 2001.

Cox, Paul. Personal communication, (1997).

Dalziel, 1937: in *Medicinal Plants in Tropical West Africa*, by Oliver Bever.

Dicks, Richard. Personal communication, 1997.

Drury, Colonel Heber. *Useful Plants of India, with Notice of Their Chief Value in Commerce, Medicine and the Arts*, 2nd edition. William H. Allen And Co. London, 1873: 296.

Duncan, S.H., Flint, H.J., and Stewart, C.S. "Inhibitory activity of gut bacteria against Escherichia coli 0157 mediated by dietary plant metabolites." *FEMS Microbiology Letter*, 164 (1998): 283-88.

"EGCg in Green Tea Found to Limit Activity of Breast Cancer Cells." *Asia Pacific Bio Tech News*, Vol. 2, Number 35, 28 Dec. 1998, p. 562.

Endocrine Today, Vol. 1, No. 3, April 2003.

Environmental Health Perspective 105(Suppl 4): 1997, pp. 977-979.

EuZhao K, Singh J. "Mechanisms of percutaneous absorption of tamoxifen by terpenes: eugenol, D-limonene and menthone." *J Controlled Release*, 1998, 55(2-3): 253-60.

Freeman, Emily and Isa Navarre. *Noni: Nature's Gift to Diabetics*, Pride Publishing: Orem, Utah, 2001.

Furusawa E, Hirazumi A, Story S, Jensen J. "Antitumour potential of a polysaccharide-rich substance from the fruit juice of Morinda citrifolia (Noni) on sarcoma 180 ascites tumour in mice." Phytother Res. 2003 Dec;17(10):1158-64.

Gary Tran, personal communication (2002).

Gerson, Scott, M.D. *Noni, Healing, and You*. Direct Source: Orem, Utah, 2001.

Giovannini M., Agostoni C., Salari P.C. "Is carnitine essential in children?" *J Int Med Res* 1991;19:88–102.

Heinicke, Ralph. *The Xeronine System*. Direct Source: Orem, Utah, 2001.

Heymsfield S.B., Allison D.B., Vasselli J.R., et al. "Garcinia cambogia (hydroxycitric acid) as a potential antiobesity agent." *JAMA* 1998;280:1596–600.

Hiramatsu, Tomonori and Masay Imoto, Takashi Koyano, Kasuo Umezawa, "Induction of Normal Phenotypes in Ras-Transformed Cells by Damnacanthal from Morinda citrifolia," *Cancer Letters*, Vol. 73, 1993.

Hirazumi, A., Rursawa, E., Chou, S.C., and Hokama, Y. "Anticancer activity of Morinda citrifolia (Noni) on intraperitoneally implanted Lewis Lung carcinoma in syngeneic mice." *Proc. West Pharmacology Society* 37 (1994): 145-46.

Hirazumi, Anne. "Anti-tumor Studies of a Traditional Hawaiian Medicinal Plant, Morinda citrifolia (Noni). In Vitro and In Vivo." Doctoral dissertation, University of Hawaii: 1997.

Hishikawa, K., Nakaki, T., Suzuki, H., Kato, R., and Saruta, T. "L-arginine as an Antihypertensive agent." *Journal of Cardiovascular Pharmacology Supplement* 20 (1992): S196-197.

Hiwasa T, Arase Y, Chen Z, Kita K, Umezawa K, Ito H, Suzuki N. "Stimulation of ultra-violet-induced apoptosis of human fibroblast UVr-1 cells by tyrosine kinase inhibitors." *FEBS Lett*. 1999 Feb 12;444(2-3):173-6.

Hohl RJ. "Monoterpenes as regulators of malignant cell proliferation." *Adv Exp Med Biol*, (1996) 401:137-46.

Hornick CA, Myers A, Sadowska-Krowicka H, Anthony CT, Woltering EA. "Inhibition of angiogenic initiation and disruption of newly established human vascular networks by juice from Morinda citrifolia (noni)." *Angiogenesis*. 2003;6(2):143-149.

"How Safe are the New NSAIDs?" *Clinician Review*, August, 1999.

http://advance.byu.edu/BYM/1999/99spring/images/superaspirin.html.

http://www.namiscc.org/Recovery/2002/NonDrugDepressionTreatments.htm

Huang, M.T., et al. Cancer Res, 1994 Feb 1; 54(3): 701-8.

Hyde, B.M., ed. The Clinical and Scientific Basis of Myalgic Encephalitis and Chronic Fatigue Syndrome. Ottawa: Nightingale Research Foundation, 1992.

K Iida VMD, K Fujita MD, H Hirai MD, H Goto MD, S Miyazaki, Y Arai MD, H Iwaki MD, M Otake MD, H Kudo MD, S Sakamoto MD. "Preventive effects of polysaccharides extracted from human tubercle bacilli (SSM; maruyama vaccine) on colonic carcinogenesis in rats," *Cancer Detection and Prevention*, 1996; 20(5).

Kamei H, et al; "Inhibition of cell growth in culture by quinones," *Cancer Biother Radiopharm*, 1998 June, 13:3, 185-8.

Kepler, A.K. Hawaiian, *Heritage Plants*. Honolulu: Oriental Publishing, 1983.

Khalsa, Dharma Singh, *The Pain Cure*. New York: Warner Books, 1999: 4-10.

Kolata, G, "Key signal of cells found to be a common gas." *The New York* Times, July 2, 1991: C1 & C6.

Krzanowski, J.J. (1996). "Chromium picolinate," *Journal of the Florida Medical Association*, 83(1), 29-31.

Kumar, et al. in *Basic Pathology*, 6th ed. W.B. Saunders Company, Philadelphia: 1997.

Levand, Oscar. "Some Chemical Constituents of Morinda citrifolia L. (Noni)." Doctoral thesis, part I, University of Hawaii; 1963: 2.

Little, Pl, et al. "A controlled trial of a low-sodium, low-fat, high-fiber diet in treated hyperensive patients: the efficacy of multiple dietary intervention." *Postgraduate Medical Journal* 66 (1990): 616-21.

Liu G, Bode A, Ma WY, Sang S, Ho CT, Dong Z. "Two novel glycosides from the fruits of Morinda citrifolia (noni) inhibit AP-1 transactivation and cell transformation in the mouse epidermal JB6 cell line." *Cancer Res*. 2001 Aug 1;61(15):5749-56.

Liu JM. et al. "Analysis of the in vitro inhibition of mammary adenocarcinoma cell adhesion by sulphated polysaccharides," *Anticancer Research*, 2000 Sep-Oct: 20(5A): 3265-71.

Lowenstein J.M. "Effect of (-)-hydroxycitrate on fatty acid synthesis by rat liver in vivo." *J Biol Chem* 1971; 246:629–32.

M.Y. Wang, W. Bender, and L.F. Yu. "Preventive Effects of Tahitian Noni Juice on the Formation of 7, 12-demethylbenz (a) anthracene (DMBA) DNA Adducts in vivo." Submitted to The American Association for Clinical Research, AACR 91st Annual Meeting: April 1-4, 2000, San Francisco.

McDougall, John A. *The McDougall Program for a Healthy Heart*. New York: Dutton, 1996: 215-16.

McKoy ML, Thomas EA, Simon OR. "Preliminary investigation of the anti-inflammatory properties of an aqueous extract from Morinda citrifolia (noni)." *Proc West Pharmacol Soc*. 2002;45:76-8.

Monica Motwani, Francis M. Sirotnak, Yuhong She, Therese Commes, and Gary K. Schwartz Drg1. "A Novel Target for Modulating Sensitivity to CPT-11 in Colon Cancer Cells." *Cancer Res*. 2002 62: 3950-3955.

Moore, T. "The role of dietary electrolytes in hypertension." *Journal of American College Nutrition* 8 (1989): 68S-80S.

Morton, Julia. "The Ocean-Going Noni, or Indian Mulberry (Morinda citrifolia) and some of Its 'Colorful' Relatives. *Economic Botany* 3 (1992): 241-256.

Mueller BA, Scott MK, Sowinski KM, Prag KA. "Noni juice (Morinda citrifolia): hidden potential for hyperkalemia?" *Am J Kidney Dis*. 2000 Feb;35(2):310-2.

Murray M.T. "The Many Benefits of Carnitine," *Am J Natural Med* 1996;3:6–14 [review].

Nakaki, T., Hishikawa, K., Suzuki, H., Saruta, T., and Kato, R. (1990): "L-Arginine-induced hypotension." *The Lancet*, 336, 696.

Newmark, Thomas M. "The Key to Fighting Inflammation." *Better Nutrition*, May 2000.

"Noni Plant May Yield New Drugs to Fight Tuberculosis," *HONOLULU*, Dec. 18, 2000. (Report of the findings at the 2000 International Chemical Congress of Pacific Basin Societies held in Honolulu, Hawaii.)

O.P. Heinonen, D. Albanes, J. Virtamo, P.R. Taylor, et al. "Prostate cancer and supplementation with alpha-tocopherol and beta-carotene: incidence and mortality in a controlled trial." *Journal of the National Cancer Institute*, 1998; 90: 440-446.

Osilesi, O., et al. "Blood pressure and plasma lipids during ascorbid acid supplementation in borderline hypertensive and normotensive adults." *Nutrition Research* 11 (1991): 405-12.

Park, K.G.M., Hayes, P.D., Garlick, P.J., Swell, H., and Eremin, O. "Stimulation of lymphocyte natural cytotoxicity by L-arginine." *The Lancet* 337 (1991): 645-646.

Personal correspondence with Jarakae Jensen, Morinda, Inc.

Personal correspondence with staff of Morinda Research Laboratory dated 8/27/01.

Phytother Res 1999 Aug; 12(5): 380-7.

Presse Med. 1955 Nov 2;63(72):1478.

Prophet, Joann M.S., R.D., "Focus On Fiber for Fitness", American Institute for Cancer Research, http://diabeticgourmet.com/articles/173.shtml.

"Psychological Symptoms in Chronic Fatigue and Juvenile Rheumatoid Arthritis," *Pediatrics* May 1999.

Ralph W. Moss, Ph.D. "New Development in Complementary Cancer Treatment." Speech to the Great Lakes College of Clinical Medicine, Inc., Baltimore, Maryland, on March 24, 2001.

Rennick et al. "Interleukin-10: an overview." *Progress in Growth Factor Research* 4 (1992): 207-227.

Rock, Joseph. "The Indigenous Trees of the Hawaiian Islands." Published under patronage; Honolulu, 1913: 467.

Salonen, J. et al. "Blood pressure, dietary fats, and antioxidants." *American Journal of American Nutrition* 48 (1988): 1226-32.

Saludes JP, Garson MJ, Franzblau SG, Aguinaldo AM. "Antitubercular constituents from the hexane fraction of Morinda citrifolia Linn. (Rubiaceae)." *Phytother Res*. 2002 Nov;16(7):683-5.

Sang S, Liu G, He K, Zhu N, Dong Z, Zheng Q, Rosen RT, Ho CT. "New unusual iridoids from the leaves of noni (Morinda citrifolia L.) show inhibitory effect on ultraviolet B-induced transcriptional activator protein-1 (AP-1) activity." *Bioorg Med Chem.* 2003 Jun 12;11(12):2499-502.

Siddiqui BS, Ismail FA, Gulzar T, Begum S. "Isolation and structure determination of a benzofuran and a bis-nor-isoprenoid from Aspergillus niger grown on the water soluble fraction of Morinda citrifolia Linn. leaves." *Nat Prod Res*. 2003 Oct;17(5):355-60.

Smith, Stephen. Globe Staff, Feb. 11, 2004.

Solomon, N. and C.C. Carpenter, I.L. Bennett and A.M. Harvey. "Schmidt's syndrome (thyroid and adrenal insufficiency) and co-existence of diabetes mellitus." *Diabetes* 14 (1965): 300.

Solomon, N.: "The Study and Treatment of the Obese Patient." *Hospital Practice*, March 1969, 4:90-94.

Solomon, Neil, and Cord Udall. *The Noni Phenomenon,* Direct Source Publishing: Vineyard, Utah, 1999.

starbulletin.com/2001/07/19/news/story11.html

"Stigma and Chronic Fatigue Syndrome." Chronic Fatigue Syndrome 5 (1999).

Sutherland, Anne. "Great ape a walking ad for all-natural arthritis relief," *Montreal Gazette*, Dec. 31, 2003.

Teitelbaum, Jacob, M.D. *From Fatigued to Fantastic!* Garden City Park, N.Y.: Avery Publishing Group/ 1996: 6.

The Journal of Rheumatology 2001; 28: 751-757.

The National Institute of Mental Health and the American Academy of Pediatrics.

"The Wealth of India." *Council of Scientific and Industrial Research* 6 (1962): 423.

Theodosakis, Jason, et al. I. New York: St. Martin's Press, 1997: 149.

Vane JR. "Inhibition of prostaglandin synthesis as a mechanism of action for aspirin-like drugs." *Nat New Biol*. 1971;231:232-235.

Vane, J.R. Inhibition of prostaglandin synthesis as a mechanism of action for aspirin-like drugs. *Nat. New Biol*. 1971; 231: 232-235.

Walsh, N.D. et al. "Analgesic Effectiveness of D-phenylalanine in chronic pain patients." *Arch Phys Med Rehabil* 7 (1986): 436-39.

Wang MY, West BJ, Jensen CJ, Nowicki D, Su C, Palu AK, Anderson G. "Morinda citrifolia (Noni): a literature review and recent advances in Noni research." *Acta Pharmacol Sin*. 2002 Dec;23(12):1127-41.

Wang, M.Y. and C. Su. "Cancer Prevention: Molecular Mechanisms to Clinical Applications," Vol. 952, 161-168. *Annals of the New York Academy of Sciences*, Dec. 2001.

Wang, Mian-Ying, M.D. "Chemopreventive Activity of Tahitian Noni Juice in C57BL-6 Mice." *UIC College of Medicine at Rockford, Dept. of Biomedical Sciences*, 1999.

Yamagami, T. "Bioenergetics in clinical medicine: Studies on coenzyme Q10 and essential hypertension." 11 (1975): 273.

Index

Abbott, Isabelle 48
abdominal breathing 113
abrasions 12
accident 12, 55, 63, 95, 105, 166
ACE inhibitors 181
acid reflux 24, 69, 238
acidophilus 142, 160
acne 89, 211, 213, 226
acupuncture 90, 231
adaptogen 38, 236
ADD 49,156-157, 224-226,
Adelaide, Barbara 173
ADHD 49, 224-227
adrenalin 219
Africa 14, 182
AIDS 54, 205-206,
alcohol 27, 41, 140, 162, 182, 228
allergies 48, 55, 84, 154, 156-158, 167,
    227, 249, 253
alpha linolenic acid 111
Alzheimer, Alois 223
Alzheimer's 21, 195-196, 223
American Association for Cancer 121, 124
amino acids 37, 43, 54, 106, 112, 142, 169,
179, 192, 194, 242, 292
analgesic 106
angina 16, 185
angioplasty 16
Ankylosing Spondylitis 99
anthraquinones 133, 144
anti-histamine 106
anti-inflammatory 21-22, 48, 70, 78, 89,
    106, 111, 130, 135, 183, 251
antibiotics 20, 78, 84, 158, 203, 242
antimicrobial 34, 44, 204
antioxidants 23, 38, 51-54, 60, 65-67,

131, 133, 141, 154, 162, 237, 239, 243
anxiety 48, 108, 152, 176, 180, 200, 217-
220, 226, 228-230
aorta 40, 187-188
apostosis 134
arginine 42, 45, 53-54, 67, 194
Armstrong, Pat 30
arteries 39-40, 54, 179, 185-189,
193, 195, 199, 240
arterioles 40-41, 187
arthritis 7, 12-13, 21-22, 26, 29-31, 33,
    59-60, 70, 74-77, 89-114, 132, 173,
    195-196, 208, 221, 223, 238
    osteoarthritis 23-24, 99, 152
asthma 75, 81, 156-158, 163, 173, 192
athlete's foot 24, 211
Australia 17, 90, 156

B-complex vitamins 142, 163
back pain 12, 95
Baggett, Robin L. 126
Ball, Tina 52
barberry root 142
Berg, Nina Elizabeth 212
beta cells 169, 171-172, 174-175, 178
beta-carotene 54, 135
beta-sitosterol 54
Bi-Polar 49
bilberry 179, 240
bladder infections 153, 205
Blobel, Guenther 66
blood pressure 7, 28, 30-31, 39, 41, 48, 59,
    67, 74-75, 77, 103, 160-161, 166, 176-
    177, 180-194, 197-201, 223, 233, 243
blood sugar 84, 165, 168-169, 171-172,
    174, 176-178, 180

boils 204-205, 211, 213
Boniek, Sharon 66, 81, 197, 214
Boykin, Michelle 2, 107
British Columbia 30
bromelain 56-60, 213-214
bronchioles 157-158, 163
Brown, Carol 80
Burma 15
bursitis 97, 99, 152

caffeine 198, 228
calcium 142, 154, 199, 229
California 63
campesterol 54
Canada 20, 72, 96, 118, 121, 149, 160
cancer 6, 13, 21, 28, 29, 30, 31, 38, 42, 44-45, 54, 59-60, 74-75, 83, 103, 115-145, 165, 190, 193, 195-196, 219, 233
candida albicans 20, 44
capillaries 40, 187
carbohydrates 167-169, 178, 228, 240, 242
carcinogens 120, 134
cardiovascular 22, 32, 40-41, 48, 67, 176, 187, 190, 193, 197, 199-201
Caribbean 95, 182
cartilage 98-99
cataracts 7, 76, 179
cat's claw 142
Ginger Caudill 224
cayenne 111, 199
celery 198
Centers for Disease Control 120, 170, 181
chamomile 111, 199
Chandler, Joan 183, 192
change in appetite 219
chemotherapy 117, 120-121, 137, 142, 144
chlamydia 44
cholesterol 28, 39, 77, 176, 180, 182-185, 195-196, 198-199, 201, 223, 233, 238, 243

chondroitin 96
chromium 66, 178, 241
chronic disease 7, 28, 35, 38, 145-164, 203
CFIDS 75, 146-149, 153-154, 163
chronic pain 6, 35, 60, 66, 74, 89-90, 92, 94-95, 97, 112-113
cigarette 78, 131
circulatory dysfunction 21
Cluley, Garry & Ingrid 92
coenzyme Q10 142, 200
coffee 27, 253
cold sores 12
colds 12, 43, 78, 203, 215
colitis 100, 155
Comfort, Betty and Neil 252
congestive heart failure 182, 184
Constantine IX 98
Cook, Leslee 63
Corbett, Tom 218
cortisol 112, 219
cough 29, 157
COX 1 enzyme 103-104, 155
COX 2 21-22, 26, 92, 100, 103-104, 113, 132-133, 155, 163, 195-196, 201, 223
COX 2 inhibitor 104, 133, 223
COX enzyme 100-101, 103, 132
cuts 12, 204

d-glucaric acid 142
Davis, Laura 149
depression 16, 48, 75, 89, 108-109, 148, 152, 154, 176, 217-231, 233
DHEA 228-229
diabetes 77, 12, 28, 31, 39, 55, 59, 66, 75, 84, 103, 146, 165 -180, 182, 233
diarrhea 28, 153, 248
Dicks, Richard 106
digestion 24, 149-150, 162, 169, 176, 179, 241

digestive problems 219
diuretics 181
dizziness 219
DL-phenylalanine 112
DNA 18, 45, 51, 119-120, 128, 130, 135
Doyle, Rich 55
dry mouth 194, 219
DuBois, Norbert M. 42
Duke University 39
Duncan, Mona 105
dye 12
dynorphins 93
dysentery 15
dysuria 15

E. coli 34, 44-45, 204, 209, 216
eczema 158, 211-212, 216
eicosapentaenoic acid 111, 179, 241
emmenagogue 15
end-stage renal disease 184
endocrine 171, 235, 238
endorphins 93, 112, 229
energy balance 149
enkephalins 93
enzymes 37, 45, 58, 65-67, 100, 103, 106,
    132, 142, 169, 179, 215, 241-242
Epigallocatechin gallate 133
erections 39
eugenol 54, 135
Europe 25, 71, 215, 229, 247
exercise 5, 27-30, 35, 70, 94, 101, 139,
    143-144, 148, 150, 152, 157, 170, 180,
    183, 188, 194, 200-201, 231, 234,
    236-237, 243

fatigue 6, 33, 76-77, 79-80, 89, 103, 147-
    148, 152-154, 165, 174, 180, 226,
    229, 254
fats 112, 141, 162, 167, 169, 178, 192,
    195, 198-199, 228

fatty acids 22-23, 111, 142, 162, 169, 179,
    199, 228, 241-242
FDA 18-19, 24-25, 57, 71, 204, 247
febrifuge 15
fennel 199
fever 15, 98-99, 137
feverfew 22-23
fiber 43, 176, 178-180, 199, 240-241
fibromyalgia 70, 75, 151-155, 163, 174
Fiji 15
fish 22, 111, 140, 154, 162, 167, 175, 178,
    195, 198-199, 228, 240-241
flavonoids 131, 179
flaxseed oil 198
Fleming, Nancie 158, 210
Florida 78, 186, 221, 234
flu 43, 78, 152, 154, 158, 203, 211
France 105-106
free radical 39, 51, 53-54, 131, 199, 239
Sigmund Freud 217
Gaby, Alan 25
gamma linolenic acid 111, 179, 241
Garcinia cambogia 241
garlic 23, 142, 163, 178, 198, 215
Gauthier, Murielle 20
germanium 142
Gerson, Scott 1, 194, 211, 216, 226
ginkgo 179, 229, 240
ginseng 23, 142, 229
glucosamine 96
glucose 149, 168-170, 176, 178-179, 234,
    240
glutamine 53-54, 67, 179, 242
glycogen 170
Golgi Apparatus 65-67, 109, 158, 192
Golgi, Camillo 65
Gotu Kola 215
gout 15, 99
Grace, Mary 190
Granby Zoo 96

Grape Seed 53, 215
green tea 215
Guam 14, 204
guarana 229
Gulf War 76
Gymnema sylvestre 179

H. pylori 17, 44, 205
Hakala, Marie 70
Hall, Steven 1, 148
Haraldsdottir, Margret 101
Harman, Denham 51
Harr, Deborah 49, 249
Hatton, Delbert 95
Hawaii 11, 14, 34, 44-45, 48, 56, 58-59,
    83, 124, 132, 191, 193, 204-205, 209
hawthorn 179, 199, 240
headaches 12, 22, 27, 48, 69, 75, 78, 93,
    147-148, 152-153, 165, 185-186, 211,
    219, 225, 238, 253
heart attack 29, 79, 181-182, 200, 219
heartbea,rapid 219

heart disease 5, 7, 16, 28-29, 75, 118,
    146, 165, 176, 181-202, 233, 243
Heinicke, Ralph 1, 56-58, 60, 62, 66-67,
    106, 108-109, 124, 213-214, 216, 220
Heller, Meria 253
hemorrhage 15
Hepatitis B 109
Herringer, Bob 23
Hettinga, Rients 225
HIV 75, 205-206
hives 158, 248
Hoerst, Joe 96
hops 200
hormones 65, 135, 149, 169, 180, 192,
    235
hunger 48, 171
hydrocortisone 79

hypericin 22
hyperkalemia 248
hypertension 40, 48, 66, 81, 181-182,
    189-190, 193-194, 197-198, 200
hypnosis 113

imagery 113
immune system 33-35, 38-44, 54, 67, 75,
    77, 98-99, 101, 106, 120-122, 124-
    127, 133, 135-137, 144, 158, 161, 163,
    171, 173-175, 181, 196, 209, 212,
    215-216
impetigo 211
India 11, 14-15, 204, 215
Indole-3 carbinol 142
Indonesia 14
infection 7, 17-18, 20, 43-44, 60, 136,
    148, 159, 196, 203-216
inflammation 22, 48, 54, 92, 94, 99-100,
    103, 111-113, 132-133, 155-157, 163,
    175, 191, 195-196, 223, 251
influenza 28
insulin 16, 39, 165, 167-172, 176-180,
    241-242
interest, loss of 219
interferon 44, 135-136, 144, 175, 209
interleukins 135-136, 175
irritability 175, 219
irritable bowel syndrome 109, 153, 160,
    187
Issell, Brian 132, 144

jaundice 15
Jensen, Jarakae 2, 104, 155
Johns Hopkins 55,172,174
Johnson, David 2, 16
Jordan, Elizabeth 63
kahunas 12, 95, 173
kava 200
kelp 142, 178

Khalsa, Dharma Singh 91
Dr. Khalsa 108
kidney 75, 130, 160-161, 165, 248
Kim, Anne Hirazumi 1, 83, 122, 124, 144, 175, 193, 209
King Saul 217
Kolodney, Samuel 1, 103
Kosinski, Terri 234, 251

L-carnitine 179, 242
Latin America 182
laxative 15
leukemia 121, 134
Levand, Oscar 45, 204
Lewis lung carcinoma 124
licorice root 215
light therapy 230-231
lignans 53-54, 67, 216
Linkroum, April 160
lipid-lowering agents 181
lipids 54, 199
lipoic acid 179
lipopolysaccharide 135-136, 175, 209
liver 15, 28, 62, 128, 130, 133-134, 142-143, 170, 216, 226, 242
Lowe, Julie 227
lupus 77, 89-90, 97, 174
lycopene 142
lymphoma 126
lymphomas 121

M. pyrogenes 204
macrophages 41-42, 44-45, 125-126, 135-136
magic bullet 21, 23, 29
magnesium 142, 154, 179, 199, 242
maitake 142
malaria 15
Malaysia 14
manganese 179, 229, 242

Marquesas Islands 12-13
Marshall, Barry 17
Martin, Gus 57
Martinez, Priscilla Salazar 239
massage therapy 231
meat 112, 140, 162, 175, 198-199, 214, 241
melatonin 48
memory 21, 39, 71, 112, 147, 153, 206, 221, 223, 229
menopause 54, 117-118, 190
menstrual 12, 15, 56, 175, 221-222
mental health 7, 217-231
metastasis 120, 134
Middle East 182
Mike, John and Susan 175
milk 37, 167, 195, 222
Missouri 227
modulate 34, 38, 135-137, 144, 175, 181, 225
monoterpenes 134, 144
Moore, Paula 203
Morinda citrifolia 55, 13, 14, 33, 85, 106, 121, 132
M. citrifolia 15
Morinda, Inc 13, 59, 71
Morton, Julia 106, 205
Moss, Ralph W. 122
multiple sclerosis 70, 75
muscle relaxation 113
muscle tension 219

naringin 179
natural killer 41-42, 135-137, 144, 175
nephritis 28
nervous system 91-92, 108, 113, 220, 229-230, 242
neurological diseases 18
neurotransmitter 48
New Guinea 18, 182

New York 5, 55, 124, 130-131, 194, 211
New Zealand 52
Nguyen, Karen 109
Nigeria 15
nitric oxide 34, 38, 40-42, 44-45, 54, 66-67, 126, 135, 144, 176, 190, 193-194, 201, 209
Nobel prize 18, 66, 100
nono 12-13
NSAIDs 100-101, 103, 105, 155
nucleotides 53, 55, 67
nutrition 5, 27-29, 66, 139, 150, 161, 178, 198, 204, 228, 233, 235, 237, 240

oats 229
obesity 75, 145, 179-180, 182, 233, 235, 237, 243
off-label 24
Oftedal, Stig 253
olive 141, 162, 198
omega-3 22-23, 228
opiates 93
osteoporosis 30, 90
ovarian tumor 117
oxidation 51, 54
oxygen 40, 51, 131, 187-188, 229

P. aeruginosa 204
Paget's 90-91
pain 7, 6, 12, 15, 20, 22, 23, 29, 33, 35, 60, 66, 70, 74, 75, 78, 89-114, 147, 151-155, 159, 163, 167, 173, 175-176, 179, 183, 185, 186, 192, 195, 197, 208, 211, 214, 221-222, 227, 238, 251, 254
pancreas 39, 133, 141, 169, 171, 174-175, 179, 241
Parkinson's 21, 75
Pau d'Arco 142
Pennsylvania 34, 230

peptide YY3-36 235
peripheral arterial disease 184
pessimism 219
phagocytes 41
Philippines 14, 205
Phosphatidyl serine 112
Phytosterols 53-54, 67, 207
Pile, Orlando 1, 166
pineapple 56, 58-60
pituitary 79
placebo 80-83, 86, 131, 194, 230
pneumonia 28
polio 28, 203
Polynesia 12-13, 15, 52, 104, 108, 155, 175
Polynesians 12, 37, 204
polyphenols 54, 131
polysaccharides 134, 144
poor circulation 176, 180
prostate 42, 133, 135, 142
proteins 37, 58, 65-67, 100, 106, 167, 169
Proteus morganii 204
proxeroninase 58, 60, 65, 67
proxeronine 37, 43, 58, 60, 62, 65-67, 158
Pruisiner, Stanley 17
Pseudomonas aeruginosa 45, 204
psychotherapy 230
Puerto Rico 14
Pycnogenol 179, 240
Pythium Sp 48

quadriplegic 55
quercetin 53-54, 67, 179

ras cells 132-133
red periwinkle 121
reishi mushrooms 142
respiratory 22, 28, 55, 75, 135, 153, 156-157, 186, 215
restlessness 219

retinopathy 176, 179
rheumatoid 98-99, 104, 111
ringworm 205, 211
Robinson, Jenna 238
Roseborough, Elizabeth 34
rosemary 199
Rosen, Jennifer 84
Rubiaceae 14
Russell, John 90

sadness 219
safety 7, 19, 24, 75, 77, 107, 111, 207, 230, 247, 249
Salmonella 44-45, 204
salt 15, 49, 141, 162, 183, 198, 249
Saludes, Jonel 207
SAM-e 229
sapraemia 15
Scanlon, Ken 159
Schanely, Gloria 221
schizandra 216
scopoletin 38, 48, 66-67, 106, 113, 176, 180, 190-192, 201, 209, 216
selenium 142, 199
serotonin 37, 48, 60, 65, 93, 108-109, 113, 219-221, 225, 228-229
shark liver 142
Shigella 45
shitake 142
Chen Shu 104, 155
Simmons, Daniel L. 103, 132
sinusitis 221
Skelly, Jan 156
skin 14, 24, 34, 48, 63, 75, 89, 101, 127, 131, 135, 153, 165, 204, 211-213, 215-216, 222, 227, 250
sleep 27, 34, 37, 48, 75, 108, 117, 147, 149, 152, 176, 186, 188, 219-221, 229-230, 237-238, 243
snake oil 19, 21-22, 25-26
snoring 23-24
sore throats 153, 215

South Pacific 6, 14
soy isoflavones 141
spastic colon 153
St. John's wort 22, 230
Stamler, Jonathan S. 39
Staphylococcus 45, 212
steroids 54, 89, 158, 186, 207
stiffness 29, 98, 101, 111, 152, 155
stigmasterol 54
Story, Stephen 12
stress 5, 17, 27, 30, 54, 75, 79, 112, 143-144, 179-180, 189, 200-201, 229-230, 241
stroke 28-29, 39, 75, 182, 184-185, 200, 219
Strommen, Leland and Alice 208
substance-P 93, 111
suicide 28
Swalling difficulty 248
swelling 95, 103, 107, 109-111, 116, 147, 149, 222, 248, 251
swollen glands 153

Tahiti 6, 11-14, 52, 118, 238
Tahitian Noni International 2, 13, 59, 71, 104-105 118, 127, 155
TAHITIAN NONI Juice 2, 25, 52-53, 71, 75, 82, 97, 105, 124, 130, 133, 155, 247-248
Taiwan 14, 105
tannins 53-54, 67
taurine 179, 242
Taylor, Chad 156
tendonitis 99, 152
terpenes 53-54, 67, 106, 113, 135, 228
terpenoid compounds 135, 144
tetrodotoxin 62
thirst 154, 172
thymus gland 54, 135
thyroid 79-80, 149
tobacco 120, 141, 162, 233, 243
toxicity 25, 71, 132, 206, 226, 248

Tran, Gary 1, 82
trigger points 153
triglycerides 54, 149
tryptophane 37
tuberculosis 28, 203, 207, 215
tumor necrosis factor 126, 135-136, 175
turmeric 111

ulcers 15, 17, 44, 100, 155, 176-177, 204-
     205, 211
United States 11-13, 25-26, 29, 71-72,
     118, 121, 146, 165, 170, 207, 223,
     227, 229, 233, 237, 243, 247
urination 15, 172
ursolic acid 54, 135
Utah 2, 49, 249

Vabekk, Inge 94
valerian 200, 230
vanadium 179, 242
Vane, John R. 100
vasoconstriction 41
vasodilation 41
venous thromboembolism 184
Vietnam 14
Virgin Islands 14
vision problems 173-174, 176
visualization 113, 138
vitamin B12 142, 179, 242
vitamin B6 142, 242
vitamin C 23, 53, 131, 141, 162, 199, 239
vitamin D 142
vitamins A and E 142, 163

Wadsworth, John 12
Wang, Mian-Ying 1, 76, 86, 128
weight control 7, 233, 241-242
West Indies 14, 204
white willow bark 112
Whiteside, Ellyn 74

Wilkinson, Clint 185
Wilson, Ann 1, 116

xeronine 37-38, 56, 58-60, 62, 66-67, 106,
     109, 213-214, 216, 220, 237

yoga 143, 231

Zamora, Phil 205
zinc 179, 229, 242
Zweifel, Doyle 160